CAN YOU HELP ME?

CAN YOU HELP ME?

INSIDE THE TURBULENT WORLD
OF HUNTINGTON DISEASE

THOMAS BIRD, MD
Professor (Emeritus), Neurology and Medical Genetics
University of Washington School of Medicine
Research Neurologist
Geriatric Research Education and Clinical Center
VA Puget Sound Health Care System
Seattle, WA

OXFORD
UNIVERSITY PRESS

OXFORD
UNIVERSITY PRESS

Oxford University Press is a department of the University of Oxford. It furthers
the University's objective of excellence in research, scholarship, and education
by publishing worldwide. Oxford is a registered trade mark of Oxford University
Press in the UK and certain other countries.

Published in the United States of America by Oxford University Press
198 Madison Avenue, New York, NY 10016, United States of America.

© Oxford University Press 2019

Library of Congress Cataloging-in-Publication Data
Names: Bird, Thomas (Thomas D.) (Neurologist), author.
Title: Can you help me? : inside the turbulent world of Huntington disease /
by Thomas Bird.
Description: New York, NY : Oxford University Press, [2019] |
Includes bibliographical references and index.
Identifiers: LCCN 2018027961 | ISBN 9780190684228 (alk. paper)
Subjects: | MESH: Huntington Disease | Case Reports
Classification: LCC RC394. H85 | NLM WL 359.5 | DDC 616.85/1— dc23
LC record available at https:// lccn.loc.gov/ 2018027961

3 5 7 9 8 6 4 2

Printed by Integrated Books International, United States of America

DEDICATION

Amelia Susman Schultz, PhD, received her doctorate in anthropology from Columbia University in 1943 (mentored by Franz Boaz and Ruth Benedict). It took 33 more years for her original dissertation to be published because it unflinchingly documented the ongoing abuse of Native American tribes in northern California. Thwarted by a career in anthropology, she moved to Seattle and in 1960 started her pioneering career as the first social worker for the new Medical Genetics Division at the University of Washington School of Medicine. In that capacity for more than 30 years she focused on assisting hundreds of families struggling with Huntington disease. Many of those families and their descendants are described in this book. In recognition of her generous personal commitment to Huntington disease, this book is dedicated to Amelia, still alive at age 103.

CONTENTS

Preface   ix

1   Introduction   1

2   Comparing Huntington Disease to Other Brain Diseases   11

3   The Genetic Testing Conundrum   21

PART I – INTERACTING WITH THE LEGAL AND MENTAL HEALTHCARE SYSTEMS

4   Can You Help Me?   33

5   It Was Awful   39

6   The Asylum   51

7   Meeting Huntington Disease Patients at Western State   63

8   I Don't Know Why I Did It   75

9   Carkeek Park   83

10   Please Call the Coroner   89

PART II – COPING STRATEGIES

11   Enjoy the Moment   95

12   High Five   103

13   Let's Try a Magnet   105

14   "I Don't Agree"   113

15   The Greatest Generation and Productive Lifestyles   121

16   Princess in Pink   127

PART III – MARRIAGE, FAMILY AND FINANCES

17 For Better, for Worse 137

18 In Sickness and in Health 143

19 Money Problems 151

20 Staying Employed 161

21 We Just Want to Have a Child 167

22 The Judge Said, "Are You Sure You Want to Do This?" 171

23 The Thanksgiving Visitor 177

24 Family Opposites 179

25 A Second Wedding 187

PART IV – EMBARRASSMENT, INJURY, NEGLECT AND DELUSIONS

26 "Excuse Me, Madam" and "I Am Not Drunk" 195

27 Broken Bones 201

28 A Bump on the Head 205

29 Impulse Control 211

30 Reservation Blues 215

31 Is This Negligence? 219

32 Delusions, Hallucinations and Diabolical Possession 225

33 The Downward Spiral 233

34 A Visit to Willow Park 239

PART V – SUMMING UP

35 Summing Up: "Can You Help Me?" 245

Acknowledgments 251
Appendix: Genetic Testing for Huntington Disease 255
Index 259

PREFACE

What is Huntington disease (HD)? It begins subtly, casually, innocently in barely noticeable little steps. Like a cat quietly stalking an unsuspecting sparrow, except often the human "sparrow" is not unsuspecting, it just has no means of escape. A quick twitch of a hand or shoulder, a little grimace that disappears. A brief loss of temper that quickly fades. Slowly, but progressively and inexorably, the disease adds symptoms and disabilities until the person ends in something like Shakespeare's last stage of humankind, sans walking, sans talking, sans swallowing and eating.

Huntington disease is a bit like Alzheimer disease, but not exactly. It is a bit like Parkinson disease, but not exactly. It is a bit like autism, bipolar disease, and schizophrenia, but not exactly. It is similar to all of these diseases, but also unique. I have seen a 5-year-old with HD and a 91-year-old with HD. This age span never happens with Alzheimer or Parkinson disease or with schizophrenia. Finally, this brain disease is absolutely genetic. Families must struggle with the knowledge that children and grandchildren are at risk for the very disease that now afflicts a loved one. Ultimately, HD is fatal, usually about 15 years after the first appearance of symptoms. Death often comes at age 55 or 45 or even 35.

Huntington disease is usually referred to as a rare degenerative disease of the brain, but it is so much more than that. One of my motivations for describing HD is personal. Over a 40+ year career I have seen more than 1,000 persons with this disease and have been constantly amazed, puzzled, distressed and impressed by the trials and tribulations of these families coping with it. Dealing with HD has been so moving, so unsettling and so challenging for me that

I felt compelled to write about it. Setting these stories down has been therapeutic for me, but I hope it will be both interesting and enlightening for you. Although HD is not common, it is also not rare. Your neighbor, coworker or family member may have HD and you are simply unaware.

Although it is uncommon, HD has medical, scientific, social and public health implications far beyond its relative infrequency in the population. It forces us to consider the relationship between the brain and thinking and behavior. It is a model for other more common brain diseases such as Alzheimer and Parkinson. It compels us to contemplate how we as individuals and communities deal with dysfunctional families and with serious mental illness.

The approach to describing HD taken in this book will be in three stages. First, there is a brief introduction to the history of HD, beginning with its identification as a clinical disease more than 140 years ago, along with an orientation regarding genetic testing for the disease and a brief description of the relevant brain anatomy. There is also a comparison of HD with other similar brain diseases. Although HD itself is relatively uncommon, its manifestations significantly overlap with those of much more common brain diseases and, therefore, its implications for our society are greatly amplified. I view HD as the canary in the mine of persons severely impaired with chronic brain diseases. What is happening to the people described in this book is also occurring on a much greater scale to those with other serious mental disturbances. All these disorders represent different ways in which the brain "disconnects."

Second, the heart of this book is a series of vignettes of patients and families struggling with the experience of HD. The vignettes will not be technical or scientific. They will show the disease as it happened in real time to real people. The extraordinary variability of the disease, its frequent anguish and occasional bright spots will be amply described. The vignettes are divided into four overlapping, but roughly distinct topics of (1) legal and incarceration issues, (2) coping strategies, (3) effects on marriage and family, and (4) difficult behavior and physical problems.

Lastly, there is a chapter dealing with the present status of treatment for HD and the encouraging research pointing toward a better future.

The vignettes you are about to read were selected from many hundreds of cases seen over more than four decades of observation. The names, places, dates and some details have often been changed for obvious reasons of privacy, but the stories are very real. Some descriptions are composites of two or three different persons.

I have attempted to collect the descriptions of these persons and their families into categories sharing common features. This has not been easy, because their stories tend to fall in a jumbled fashion from my memory and each tale had unique aspects. It sometimes seems as if they are photographs falling from a family album, the HD family album. I have tried to organize the material as carefully as possible. My mind often generates a detailed image of these patients and their family members as if they have returned to tell their stories. The chapters in this book will show the tremendous variety of experiences that color and shape HD as it moves through a family.

Many of the case histories described in this book will be frustrating, depressing or even disturbing to read. This is partly because the practice of medicine sometimes resembles the complaint desk at a department store. The patients we see are heavily skewed toward unhappy, frustrated persons in distress who sometimes represent disasters in the making. Furthermore, we obviously tend to remember the most dramatic cases from this skewed group. Nevertheless, as you will see, HD is a terrible and devastating disease such that disturbing examples are not difficult to find. Suggesting otherwise or ignoring such cases would be sugar-coating the disease. That said, I have made a concerted effort to describe many persons with HD who have lived successful and rewarding lives, have maintained an impressive optimistic outlook, and whose families have demonstrated superb coping abilities.

I still vividly recall the first two patients with a diagnosis of HD I saw nearly 50 years ago. They were both men in their 30s or 40s who had been admitted to the Neurology ward of the Seattle VA Medical Center when I was a neurology resident in training. The first man had frequent jumpy, jerky movements of his body that he could not control, and he was suspicious and reluctant to talk about his family and his past experiences. I can still picture him in his thin, blue hospital bathrobe looking worried and frightened. He stands out in my mind because I subsequently cared for his son and two grandsons, all of whom eventually developed the disease. The genetic burden for their family was inescapable. It was agonizing to watch three generations of this family repeatedly battered by this disease. I can still feel the intense sadness and frustration of dealing with their continuing predicament.

The second man had even worse involuntary movements that especially involved his face and tongue. He constantly carried a white cotton napkin in his mouth to absorb saliva and to prevent injury to his lips and tongue from his chewing movements. His sad visage still haunts me. He also stands out in my mind because several years later we discovered that his diagnosis of HD was actually an error. He was found to have odd, spiny-shaped red blood cells that were a clue to a different diagnosis. He had a genetic brain disease that closely masqueraded as HD but was quite different at the molecular level. In fact, it was a recessive rather than dominant genetic disease, and his children were not at risk for his ultimately fatal condition. This man impressed upon me the great importance of being certain about the accurate diagnosis of HD. He also made me realize that genetic diseases of the brain were going to be more complicated, more puzzling and more fascinating than I had ever imagined.

I had no idea at the time that these two patients were starting me on a 40+ year journey interacting with hundreds of families trying to cope with HD. Their stories are the core of this book. William Carlos Williams, who was both a poet and a physician, said that a doctor could and should spend most of a career just listening to patients. That is what I have tried to accomplish with these families. The following pages reflect what I have heard.

■ ■ ■

The poem springs from the half-spoken words of such patients as the physician sees from day to day. He observes it in the peculiar, actual conformations in which life is hid. Humbly he presents himself before it and by long practice he strives as best he can to interpret the manner of its speech. In that the secret lies. This, in the end, comes perhaps to be the occupation of the physician after a lifetime of careful listening.

—WILLIAM CARLOS WILLIAMS

1

Introduction

BRIEF HISTORY OF HUNTINGTON DISEASE

The disease we now call Huntington (HD) has undoubtedly been around for centuries. It was probably first thought to be a mental illness, or perhaps caused by a stroke, or even possession by the devil. The abnormal body movements were sometimes called "St. Vitus' dance" (named for the patron saint of dancing) and that, in turn, was a term used to label children who developed jerky movements in the early stages of rheumatic fever. In 1806, 40-year-old Phoebe Hedges, of East Hampton, Long Island, was overcome by this disease and drowned herself in the Atlantic Ocean.[1] She was a member of the original American family, subsequently described in 1872 by Dr. George Huntington, a 22-year-old Long Island general physician who had watched this strange family for many years as his physician father and grandfather cared for them over many decades (Figure 1.1).

The involuntary movements like those seen in Phoebe Hedges were originally called "chorea" because they resembled dancing or choreography. The disturbing combination of unexpected movements and dysfunctional behavior often resulted in the families being shunned by their neighbors and communities even though intelligence was not affected. George Huntington briefly and accurately described the main features of the disease in 1872, namely the adult onset of abnormal, involuntary movements of the arms, legs and face coupled with problems affecting thinking and behavior, which he termed "a tendency to insanity." He noted the disease occurred in both men and women, was progressive and shortened lifespan. In his 19th-century prose he prophetically said of the disease, "Once it begins it clings to the bitter end

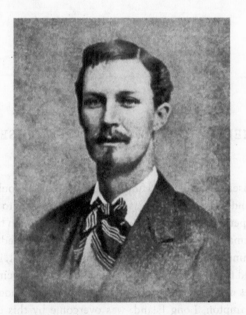

Figure 1.1 ■ Dr. George Huntington, who in 1872, at age 22, wrote the earliest description of the disease that bears his name. He carefully observed a family with hereditary chorea living in East Hampton, Long Island, that had been patients of his father and grandfather.

until the hapless sufferer is but a quivering wreak of his former self."[2] He noted that it was inherited, passed along by either fathers or mothers, but if a family member lived to advanced age without showing signs of the disease, the offspring of that person escaped the condition and that branch of the family remained forever free. Huntington was also well aware of the role played by depression and suicide in these families, which will become an important theme later in this book.

In the mid-20th century there was speculation that early American colonists with HD had been persecuted as witches. This speculation turned out to be entirely false, but it added to the stigma of the disease at that time. Huntington disease was one of the "undesirable conditions," such as alcoholism, mental retardation and criminality, which the American eugenicists of the 1920s and 1930s hoped to eliminate from the population by sterilization. Much of this eugenics analysis was done by Dr. Elizabeth Muncey under the direction of Charles Davenport. Davenport had established the Record Office of the Cold Spring Harbor Laboratory on Long Island, ironically only a few miles from East Hampton, the home of Phoebe Hedges and George Huntington. This eugenics theme was easily incorporated into the extermination programs of the Nazis in Germany where HD was included in the category of "lives not worth living."

Although often considered "rare," there are plenty of people with HD. This is especially important considering the severity of the disease. There are no exact numbers, but it is estimated that in the United States there are between 30,000 and 50,000 symptomatic persons with HD and 120,000–150,000 of their family members are at genetic risk for the disease. In Washington state there are at least 600–700 people with symptomatic HD and more than 2,000–3,000 family members at risk.

HUNTINGTON DISEASE MIGRATION

The first families with HD in this country came from Northern Europe and settled in New England and New York. Now, several centuries later, a study based on death certificates suggests that the state of Washington had two to three times as many persons with HD as numerous other states. This was also true of California and Oregon. How did this happen? At first we thought this might be the result of a "founder effect," which would result from a single person with HD moving to the Pacific Northwest more than 100 years ago; we would now be seeing the descendants of that individual. We quickly realized that this was not the case, because careful inspection of our patients' family pedigrees revealed they were from unrelated, separate families. More likely, the large number of families with HD in the Pacific Northwest is the result of a sociological migration pattern. Migration is not random. People who pick up and leave home are different from people who stay put. Migrants move on for many different reasons. Some are loners, uncomfortable with society, while others are viewed as "different" and subtly, or not so subtly, ostracized. Historically in our country those kinds of individuals tended to move west. I think that is what has happened to many persons with HD, and they have literally piled up on the West Coast. I have no better explanation.

Of local historical interest, David Johnson (an amateur Seattle genealogist with a family connection to HD) has discovered that the first person in the Pacific Northwest with the HD-associated gene was a relative of Phoebe Hedges, "the woman who walked into the sea" in 1806. She was a member of the original Long Island family with HD studied by George Huntington. Her grandson, Hiram, came to the Northwest over the Oregon Trail in the 1850s. The reason for his pulling up stakes in the East and making the arduous trek to the far West are unknown. Perhaps he was restless, agitated or even delusional. Perhaps he was ostracized by his community. We will never know. In any event, one of his descendants ended up in the Oregon State Mental Hospital, in the state capitol, Salem.

THE HUNTINGTON GENE AND
THE GENETIC TEST

In the second half of the 20th century HD became a model for the scientific study of genetic diseases. The location of the gene for the disease was discovered in 1983 by a collaborative team of scientists influenced strongly by the work of Nancy Wexler, a psychologist who was herself at risk for HD. This project studied a village in Venezuela populated by a large family containing dozens of people with HD. Ten years later, in 1993, the gene for HD was identified by the same scientists. For families with HD and physicians caring for them the most important aspect of the HD gene discovery was the rapid availability of a simple DNA-based blood test for the presence or absence of the molecular abnormality in the gene. Prior to this discovery persons at 50% risk of HD, because they had an affected parent and this is an autosomal dominant genetic disease, simply had to wait and watch to see whether or not they developed symptoms of the disease. This watchful waiting was the only method to determine whether a person had inherited it. It was never certain how long they had to wait, but it was generally thought they had to at least make it to age 60 without symptoms before they could feel they had "escaped." But in 1993, with the discovery of the HD gene, there was finally a test that could answer the genetic risk question at any age. The problem then became, did family members want to know? Because it is a terrible disease and there is no specific treatment or prevention, most family members were wary of being tested. An important minority of family members, however, do proceed with testing. The repercussions, the "fallout," are described in the vignettes of Chapter 3.

Because genetic testing is so important in today's HD world, a few related points are made here to better understand the genetic test results mentioned in the next chapters. For interested readers, more specific details regarding genetic testing, along with an explanatory figure, can be found in the Appendix.

- The genetic test measures the size of a stretch of DNA in the huntingtin gene, called a *CAG expansion*.
- The test result is a number delineating how many CAG repeats are found in this expansion.
- A "normal" (or "negative") test result means 27 or fewer CAG repeats were found in the gene, indicating that the individual has not inherited the DNA variant associated with HD.
- An "abnormal" or "positive" test result means 40 or more CAG repeats were found. A person with this result will develop symptoms of HD if he or she lives a normal lifespan.

- 27 to 34 CAG repeats is considered an "intermediate" range, which is described in more detail in the Appendix.
- 35 to 39 CAG repeats is called the range of "reduced penetrance" and may be associated with late age of onset (after age 60).
- A test result of 60 or more CAG repeats is often associated with early onset of HD symptoms, frequently in the juvenile-onset ages (before age 20). When the result is greater than 80 the onset is often before age 10.
- In general, the test result does NOT indicate the precise age of onset of symptoms nor the type of symptoms the individual will experience.

THE BRAIN ANATOMY OF HUNTINGTON DISEASE

The gene associated with HD (called the *HTT* gene) contains chemical information (a "code") that tells the cell to make a protein called huntingtin. The exact function of this protein remains unclear, but it certainly is necessary for the normal activity of many brain cells. When the *HTT* gene contains too many CAG repeats (more than 30 or 40) it codes for a huntingtin protein that is misshapen and no longer functions properly. The brain cells that use this protein are no longer able to perform activities correctly and they slowly deteriorate over a period of many months and years. This is the cause of the deterioration of nerve cells occurring in the brains of persons with HD.

In terms of anatomy, the abnormal protein produced by the genetic mutation in HD does not equally damage all regions of the human brain. Hardest hit is a relatively small region deep within the brain known as the *striatum of the basal ganglia* (Figure 1.2). Within this region the greatest damage occurs in an area called the *caudate nucleus*. There are a collection of nerve cells within the caudate called *medium spiny neurons*, and they seem to be especially vulnerable to the abnormal HD protein. Shrinkage (atrophy) of the caudate is sometimes seen on computed tomography (CT) or magnetic resonance (MRI) brain images, especially in persons with symptomatic HD

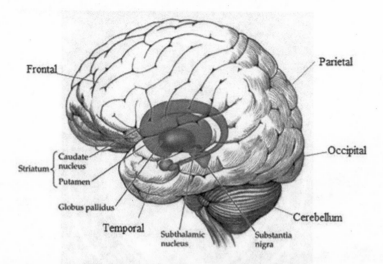

Figure 1.2 ▪ A group of nuclei deep in the center of the brain are termed the basal ganglia, which includes the striatum. The nerve cells in the caudate nucleus in the striatum are particularly hard hit in Huntington disease, and the substantia nigra is involved in Parkinson disease. The caudate has direct connections to the frontal lobe as well as to other areas of the cerebral cortex.

(Figure 1.3). The basal ganglia has several different functions, but a major function is coordination and integration of body movements. Thus, it is not surprising that damage to this region produces both uncoordinated and involuntary movements (chorea). However, the brain damage caused by HD is more extensive than just in the basal ganglia. The connections to the cerebral cortex and the cortex itself also undergo deterioration (a kind of "disconnection"). This is especially true of the connections to the frontal lobes. The damage to the basal ganglia and its cortical connections likely underlies the poor judgement, personality changes, and other aberrations of thinking and behavior that occur in people with HD.

The mutation causing HD is in all cells of the person who has inherited it, not just in brain cells. How it may cause dysfunction in cells outside the brain is not entirely clear and is the focus of considerable

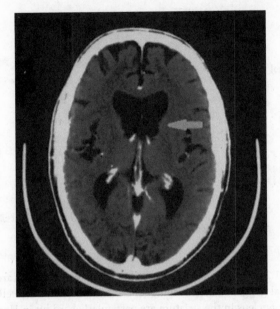

Figure 1.3 ■ MRI image of the brain in a patient with Huntington disease demonstrating shrinkage (atrophy) of the caudate (arrow).

research. The abnormal protein seems to disturb mitochondria (commonly called the "energy batteries" of the cell) and may be related to the fact that persons with HD are rarely obese, have trouble maintaining weight, and also sometimes have difficulty regulating body temperature. The reader wishing to learn more about the scientific basis of HD is referred to several excellent and detailed reviews of this topic by Bates, Tabrizi, Hayden, and their colleagues.[2,3]

THE SYMPTOMS OF HUNTINGTON DISEASE

Huntington disease is usually divided into three overlapping clinical manifestations: motor, cognitive, and behavioral. The *motor* part refers to involuntary, adventitious movements (chorea) of hands, face, feet or the whole body that can be socially embarrassing and lead to incoordination and clumsiness. The *cognitive* piece often presents as difficulties with problem solving and making correct decisions. The *behavioral* component is the most variable and can include impaired judgment, poor impulse control, obsessive/compulsive disorder, apathy or agitation, and even occasionally delusions and hallucinations. Furthermore, depression is common, as is a lack of insight, often appearing as a lack of awareness of one's own disabilities. In my experience, roughly speaking, about one third of persons begin to show signs of the disease with just motor symptoms, about one third begin with just cognitive/behavioral problems, and about one third began with a combination of all three. In the advancing stages of the disease most persons will eventually exhibit all components of the disease, but some continue to primarily show only one of the major symptoms. Although HD is rightly considered a "movement disorder" because of the frequent and readily apparent involuntary jerks and twitches, it is the behavior and cognitive problems that become most frustrating and disabling for the affected persons and their families.[4] In the last months or even years of the disease the affected person is often confined to bed, unable to walk or talk, and completely dependent for their every need on a family member or healthcare professional.

It is not easy to fully describe chorea. A picture is worth a thousand words, or, in this case, a film. I have seen a short, silent movie made 60 years ago that shows a remarkable example of chorea. I call it "The Smoker." A man with HD sits on a small chair staring off to his right. His face is busy with movements: a smile, then a frown; eyebrows up, eyebrows down. A cigarette dangles from his lips, always on the verge of falling, but does not. He crosses and uncrosses his knees, leans forward, then back, then to his left. His arm darts off to the right, then arches back as he deftly snatches the cigarette from his mouth, followed by his arm with the cigarette between his fingers abruptly changing direction and now pointing directly at the camera, as if offering a smoke to the viewer. In a few seconds, his head tips back, he pops the cigarette back in his mouth and the whole process repeats, but with a slightly different combination of movements. Watching him perform this simple task is mesmerizing. He appears to have two different nervous systems operating simultaneously in parallel: one jerky, unpredictable and uncoordinated, the other surprisingly accurate and on target. This is the chorea of HD in action.

PLACING HUNTINGTON DISEASE IN MEDICAL CONTEXT

Huntington disease is certainly not the only disorder in which the brain slowly degenerates and "disconnects." In fact, many similar diseases are much more common than HD. The next chapter will briefly show how these various diseases overlap, how they are like and unlike HD, and help the reader put HD into context within the larger world of degenerative brain diseases.

References

1. Wexler, Alice. *The Woman Who Walked into the Sea.* Yale University Press, New Haven, 2008.
2. Bates GP, Tabrizi S, Jones L. *Huntington's Disease,* 4th ed. Oxford University Press, New York, 2014.
3. Bates GP, Dorsey R, Gusella JF, Hayden MR, Kay C, Leavitt BR, Nance M, Ross CA, Scahill RI, Wetzel R, Wild EJ, Tabrizi SJ. Huntington disease. *Nature Reviews. Disease Primers,* 1:15005, 2015.
4. Simpson J, Lovecky D, Kogan J, Vetter L, Yohrling G. Survey of the Huntington's disease patient and caregiver community reveals most impactful symptoms and treatment needs. *Journal of Huntington's Disease,* 5:395–403, 2016.

2

Comparing Huntington Disease to Other Brain Diseases

When I first started seeing patients with Huntington disease I expected certain "classic" symptoms and a predictable downhill trajectory. I expected involuntary movements and impulsive behavior followed by dementia and death over a 15-year period. Looking back on more than a thousand patients with this disease, I am astonished by the variability I have seen. Perhaps this simply confirms that every individual is unique and that I have seen so many individuals "up close and personal," but it's more than that. The manifestations have been highly idiosyncratic and unpredictable. Some persons have chorea, and some do not. In those with the movements the chorea can be mild and of little consequence. In others, the jerks and twitches can progress to a serious disability impeding walking, causing frequent falls and requiring a wheelchair. Some patients have disturbing delusions, but most do not. Obsessive-compulsive behavior is fairly common, but absent in many. One person may be agitated, impulsive and unpredictable. The next will be an apathetic couch potato. A child may have symptoms at age 5 and die at 12, whereas someone else is happily retired and still driving at 75. There are people with HD who have been successful doctors, lawyers, engineers and college professors, balanced by others who have found it impossible to maintain any kind of employment. Every instance of this disease has had its surprises and unexpected turn of events. I have sometimes felt like the private eye Kinsey Milhone in Sue Grafton's alphabet mysteries, sitting by my phone, wondering if the next call will be from a public defender, prosecuting attorney, parole officer, or coroner.

As you read this book you will experience this variety: from prisons and homicide to Texas line dancing and money hidden in a shoe; from suicide and subdural hematomas to preimplantation diagnosis in an embryo; from asylums and electroconvulsive therapy (ECT) to diabolic possession; from teachers, to lawyers, to truck drivers.

This remarkable variability in the manifestations of HD is one of the most puzzling aspects of the disease. The dozens of people described in this book are a testimony to that extreme variety. This phenomenon is different from most other degenerative brain diseases. Everyone with Alzheimer disease has memory loss and it is always progressive. Everyone with Parkinson disease develops stiffness and rigidity and it progressively worsens. This is not to say that there is no individual variability in Alzheimer and Parkinson diseases. Of course there is, but there are simply no symptoms of HD that are always present or that always progress. It is unknown what biological aspects of HD send the brain off in inappropriate misdirected paths and what factors modify how and when this happens. A small enlargement of a particular part of DNA produces a slightly abnormal protein which in turn somehow begins a slow cascade of disconnections in the brain. Understanding the modifiers and influencers of these processes would tell us a great deal about the biological drivers of human behavior. We are a long way from that understanding.

Another difficult problem has always been trying to judge "when the disease begins," usually meaning when the first symptoms appear. Traditionally, that always meant the first signs of the involuntary movements. That in itself can be problematic because the early movements are so subtle. An experienced clinician can get quite good at noticing the twitches at an early stage and differentiating them from simple nervousness or habit twitches. Later in the disease they can become obvious, representing a so-called "metro bus diagnosis," noticeable to any passenger (like "the smoker" described in the Introduction). But what about the patients who develop movements late in the disease or never? When does their disease "begin"? In these persons it is the cognitive or behavior changes that are the first to appear. These can be difficult to distinguish from anxiety, stress, depression or normal personality quirks. Yet, there is no doubt that the earliest signs can be episodic loss of temper control, unexpected and bizarre statements, new compulsions or obsessions, shortened attention span, or lapses in judgment, especially regarding finances. Of course, the abnormal gene mutation is inherited at conception and presumably at work in the brain from the very beginning of development. Detailed MRI brain scans have shown anatomical signs of the disease a decade before the first noticeable clinical symptoms. Nevertheless, there clearly are people with the mutated gene who have many decades of happy, successful lives before developing the first signs. Furthermore, some individuals succumb to the disease in less than a decade, whereas others survive with symptoms for more than 25 years. So little time, so much to learn.

▪ ▪ ▪

ALZHEIMER DISEASE

It helps to compare HD with other more common degenerative diseases of the brain. For example, Alzheimer disease (AD) was first recognized as a unique brain disorder by Dr. Alois Alzheimer, in 1907. More than 100 years later it is now regarded as the most common degenerative brain disease. The hallmark of AD is a kind of dementia that early and prominently involves a loss of memory. This is a major difference with Huntington. Persons with HD often have quite good memories and, for that reason alone, would not be confused with the typical person with AD. Patients with HD may have poor judgment, short attention span and impulsive behavior, but they recognize their friends and family and can tell you where they are and what they had for breakfast. Not so with AD. However, similar to HD, people with AD commonly have a lack of awareness about the severity of their memory loss and often their more extensive confusion and disorientation. Furthermore, patients with AD often have language impairment not seen in HD. Also, patients with AD do not develop chorea. The brain pathology in AD starts in two regions, called the *hippocampus* and the *parietal lobe*, and slowly spreads throughout the entire cerebral cortex. The pathology in HD begins in a very different region deep in the brain (the caudate or striatum) and spreads in a different manner. Also, although both diseases are slowly progressive over a period of years, people with AD often die within 8 to 10 years of their first symptoms whereas those with HD usually live much longer. In addition, although there are genetic factors influencing the risk of developing AD, most AD is not strictly genetic in the way that HD is. Intriguingly, we have seen several persons with HD who have gone on to also develop AD. Their HD symptoms merged into the severe progressive memory loss and confusion of AD. Nothing says that an occasional individual cannot develop two brain diseases. The resulting dementia is completely incapacitating.

An exception is a rare form of AD referred to as familial early-onset AD. This type represents not more than 2% of all AD, but the genetic factor works just like that in HD. That is, this early-onset form of AD shows autosomal dominant inheritance, and each child of an affected person is at 50% risk, just as in HD. This form of AD usually has the onset of dementia in the 40s and 50s, sometimes as early as the 30s. The memory loss and confusion are severely progressive over 4 to 5 years, causing great distress to the families and resulting in a bedridden state and death in less than 10 years. These families experience many of the distresses and disruptions seen in families with HD. A striking example is the family with AD in which persons with the disease have "the thousand mile stare," a sustained blank expression seen in many degenerative brain diseases, including HD.[1]

■ ■ ■

FRONTOTEMPORAL DEMENTIA

Another less well-known brain disease that has many similarities with HD is termed frontotemporal dementia, or FTD. This condition usually develops in the 40s and 50s and has many of the behavioral and cognitive characteristics of HD, such as lack of impulse control, agitation or apathy, and unexpected antisocial behaviors, all occurring in the context of intact memory function. Many types of FTD are also inherited in an autosomal dominant genetic pattern just like in HD. Lack of awareness can be extreme in FTD. I once saw a patient with FTD who would crawl around the floor of department stores looking for loose change and thought this was a perfectly normal activity. As the name implies, this disease predominantly affects the frontal and temporal lobes of the brain, correlating with the abnormal behaviors. Over the years, I have been struck with the many similarities between FTD and HD. Persons with FTD can fall through the cracks in society and become homeless, just like individuals with HD. For example, a national award–winning librarian in New York City developed symptoms later recognized as FTD, including serious financial mismanagement (we'll see similar stories in Chapter 19). His life ended with the same fate as the HD patient we will meet in Chapter 8: both men became homeless and vulnerable and were murdered by their roommates over trivial arguments.[2] Just as with HD, the genetic forms of FTD and early-onset familial AD have diagnostic blood tests available to family members, who must decide whether or not they want to learn their genetic status.[3]

▪ ▪ ▪

PARKINSON DISEASE

Parkinson disease (PD) is another common neurodegenerative disorder. It was first described in England in the 18th century by Dr. James Parkinson. People with PD have an abnormal movement, namely a regular resting tremor of their hands. Overall, however, they become extremely slow to move. Walking, eating and dressing eventually take an inordinate amount of time. Although persons with PD often develop trouble with their memory and confusion late in the disease, they rarely experience the impulsivity, agitation and unexpected behaviors seen in people with HD. However, an interesting aspect of PD is that side effects resulting from its best treatment, the drug L-dopa, can actually cause chorea and sometimes obsessive-compulsive behavior, such as gambling addiction. Persons with PD usually live much longer than those with HD, and PD primarily affects a different part of the brain, namely the substantia nigra. Also, most PD is not genetic, although, just as with AD, there are genetic variants of PD.

■ ■ ■

AMYOTROPHIC LATERAL SCLEROSIS

Amyotrophic lateral sclerosis, also known as ALS or Lou Gehrig's disease, manifests primarily as progressive weakness. The weakness can start in the arms or legs or tongue, but eventually it spreads throughout the entire body. The disease is more rapidly progressive than HD and persons with ALS rarely live more than two or three years, with a few dramatic exceptions. Late in the disease there may be cognitive deficits, but not the significant behavioral changes often seen in HD or the dementia of AD. Most persons with ALS do not have a genetic disease, but just as with AD and PD, there are definite genetic subtypes of ALS. Obviously, an autosomal dominant genetic form of ALS is devastating to the families.

■ ■ ■

CREUTZFELDT-JACOB DISEASE

The rarest of the degenerative brain diseases is called Creutzfeldt-Jacob disease (CJD), named after the two German physicians who first described it. Its prevalence in the population is about one to two cases per million, so most doctors have never seen a case. It causes severe shaking tremors, muscle rigidity and dementia, with death often within less than two or three years. Similar to AD, PD, and ALS, most occurrences are not inherited, but 10–15% are definitely genetic. The disease is caused by a small misfolded protein called a prion. In the sporadic cases the disease can be transmitted by direct tissue contact or transplant and is responsible for "mad cow disease." The genetic form is inherited in an autosomal dominant fashion, just like in HD, and there is a genetic test for mutations in the prion gene. Gina Kolata has written a clear history of the "discovery" of CJD and a moving description of its tremendous impact on an affected family.[4]

Another commonality among the various degenerative brain diseases is that, at the biochemical level, many of them show deposition or aggregation of a specific protein in or around the nerve cells. In HD the protein is huntingtin. In AD the proteins are amyloid and tau. In PD the aggregating protein is alpha synuclein, and in many cases of FTD and ALS there is deposition of a protein called TDP-43, and also tau in some cases of FTD. In CJD the protein is prion. The mechanisms initiating and regulating these protein aggregations are important therapeutic targets in each of the diseases and could even overlap between diseases.

■ ■ ■

TOURETTE SYNDROME

There are several similarities between HD and Tourette syndrome (TS). Persons with TS have involuntary movements (tics) and often obsessive-compulsive symptoms and there is an incompletely described genetic component. However, TS usually begins in childhood, the tics are most commonly facial and vocal, and the condition often improves with age. Nevertheless, persons with TS are occasionally misdiagnosed as having HD and vice versa.

■ ■ ■

BIPOLAR DISORDER

Depression is very common in HD, occurring in approximately 40–50% of persons with the disease at some point in their lifetime. Some of the depression is likely a reaction to dealing with the disease, but there is evidence that the disease itself can cause depression. It is one of the symptoms associated with HD that is amenable to treatment, such as psychotherapy or antidepressant medication. Episodes of mania are much less common in HD but certainly occur and may have been present in Woody Guthrie, whom we will meet in Chapter 6. In the general population, when depression and mania alternate in the same individual it has been called manic-depressive illness or bipolar disorder. This condition is estimated to be present in about 1–2% of the general population. The depression can be profound, the mania can be out of control, and the disorder can be disabling and devastating. One of the most compelling descriptions of bipolar disorder is the biography of the American poet Robert Lowell, written by Kay Redfield Jameson.[5] Lowell experienced multiple admissions to mental hospitals, ECT treatment, and numerous medications. Yet, he was convinced that the disease contributed to his impressive creativity. The disorder also has a strong genetic component, as exemplified by the family histories of both Robert Lowell and Ernest Hemingway. No single gene or consistent combination of genes has been identified as directly causative. Unlike HD, bipolar disorder is not strictly degenerative. However, the illness has long episodes of mania lasting weeks or months that cycle with prolonged periods of depression. The biological basis of these long cycles is unknown.

■ ■ ■

SCHIZOPHRENIA

Finally, several of the behavioral characteristics of HD are reminiscent of schizophrenia. As noted in this book, there are a few patients with HD who experience delusions and auditory hallucinations highly similar to those seen in schizophrenia (known as "positive" symptoms).

In fact, I have seen patients with HD who initially were diagnosed as having schizophrenia. This has happened too often to be passed off as a coincidence. Schizophrenia is undoubtedly a brain disease. Although it does not have the dramatic neuropathological hallmarks of HD, AD, PD or FTD, schizophrenia is unquestionably due to abnormalities of brain biochemistry and physiology. Its frequent improvement with chemicals that alter brain biochemistry emphasizes this point. It is likely that the frontal lobes and the basal ganglia are dysfunctional in people with schizophrenia, just as they are in persons with HD and FTD. Schizophrenia also has strong genetic factors at play, but it is not inherited in an autosomal dominant fashion like HD.[6]

The personal and social disability caused by schizophrenia is surprisingly variable. In addition to "positive" symptoms, patients with both schizophrenia and HD may experience "negative" symptoms, such as apathy, poor attention and social withdrawal. Many persons are so disturbed that they are unable to function in any reasonable manner and may be resistant to treatment. Others, while episodically impaired and requiring medication, are not only functional but even highly successful and productive. Elyn Saks wrote a revealing book about her battle with the disease and became a professor of law, psychology, and psychiatry and the behavioral sciences at UCLA.[7] This variability of psychotic features can also be seen in HD.

Dr. Saks' story is especially poignant in describing the ambivalence patients feel toward their antipsychotic medications. They feel well when taking medicine, but sometimes have unwanted side effects like drowsiness or apathy. Since they feel so "normal" while taking medication, they decide they can stop taking the pills and within a few days become disturbingly psychotic. It's a cycle that is hard to break, and can also happen in HD. Persons with HD often refuse to take medication that really seems to be helping them, because they "feel fine."

This brief trip through the world of neurodegenerative diseases highlights the point that HD is actually unique. There is no other condition quite like it. However, its many overlapping characteristics with these more common brain diseases strongly imply that a better understanding of HD will also lead to an improved understanding of its neurological relatives, and vice versa.

References

1. Reiswig G. *The Thousand Mile Stare: One Family's Journey Through the Struggle and Science of Alzheimer's*. Nicholas Brealey, London, 2010.
2. Peltz J. The awful odd downfall of the school librarian of the year. Associated Press, New York, April 10, 2017.
3. For more information on FTD see http://www.theaftd.org.
4. Kolata G. *Mercies in Disguise*. St. Martin's Press, New York, 2017.
5. Jamison KR. *Robert Lowell, Setting the River on Fire: A Study of Genius, Mania, and Character*. Knopf, New York, 2017.
6. Cohen B. *Theory and Practice of Psychiatry*. Oxford University Press, New York, 2003.
7. Saks E. *The Center Cannot Hold: My Journey Through Madness*. Hachette Books, New York, 2007.

The Genetic Testing Conundrum

Some people don't like the term *counseling*. It sounds too much like psychotherapy, and they are wary of that. In fact, genetic counseling does sometimes have a heavy dose of psychotherapy, but it entails much more. Perhaps the best single word would be *education*—genetic education. Trained genetic counselors primarily address four basic questions: How can the genetic diagnosis be documented? What are the characteristics of this genetic disease? What are my risks and the risks to other family members of inheriting the disease? What strategies are available for dealing with this disease in my family and dealing with my risk for it?

For Huntington disease the education includes a description of a typical case with onset in the 40s, slow progression, and death in the 50s. The ends of the age spectrum are also described, including juvenile cases at one end and late onset after the age of 60 or 70 at the other. The involuntary motor movements and the cognitive behavioral changes are noted. The availability of treatments for certain symptoms such as the movements, depression and agitation are mentioned, but the lack of a drug to prevent, halt or reverse the disease must be explained. And the key genetic feature is that each child, male or female, of a person with the disease stands at 50% risk to inherit the genetic mutation from that parent.

During counseling the range of test results is described, including clearly normal, clearly abnormal, and the so-called gray range, where one may or may not develop symptoms of HD (see Appendix for more details). The pros and cons of testing are discussed. A negative (normal) test may relieve anxiety. A positive (abnormal) test may worsen anxiety. A positive test does not affect the ability to obtain health insurance, but it could adversely affect the ability to obtain life, disability or long-term care insurance. Remember, as described in Chapter 1, a positive test result in this context means the laboratory has identified the DNA variant or mutation associated with HD. It does not mean the person has symptoms of HD, nor can the result accurately predict when symptoms will develop. It only means the individual has inherited the HD-associated variant (mutation) from one of the parents.

The reasons why someone is seeking genetic testing also need to be explored. The most common motivation is often a kind of persistent, unremitting curiosity that can only be resolved by knowing the result. One must also consider who else will be told the test result and what they will do with that information. Will a positive test result reduce your chances of getting a job, being an airline pilot, joining the army, or being a school teacher? Of the thousands of persons at risk for HD, only a small fraction decide to proceed with and complete genetic testing. The vast majority of persons at risk would rather not know their genetic result, since a test showing the mutation can be depressing, and there is no means of prevention. Whether the test is positive or negative, the family needs to hear that there will always an experienced, compassionate team to help them through this challenge.

Knowing whether or not you would want genetic testing if you were at risk for a hereditary brain disease is a tough question to answer.

Before the gene associated with HD was identified, that is, when genetic testing was "theoretical," about 75% of persons at risk for the disease said that they would want genetic testing. Now that the test is actually available, no more than 10% of persons at risk choose to be tested. Although cost and matters of privacy may play a role, many other reasons for this change in attitude have become apparent.

For patients and physicians there are two major considerations for getting a genetic test for HD. The first is for an individual who has no symptoms but is at 50% risk because of an affected parent. A positive test result will indicate that the person has inherited the mutation causing HD, but symptoms may not occur for years or even decades. The stories about to be related in this chapter fall into that category. The second reason for testing is for persons who are already showing symptoms—the test result is used to confirm the clinical diagnosis. This is the testing situation that is described in most of the later chapters. Lisa Genova has dealt thoughtfully with these testing scenarios in her novels about HD and familial Alzheimer disease.[1,2]

Inaccurate genetic information can be confusing and, sometimes, seriously misleading. Woody Guthrie, perhaps America's most famous folk singer, knew his mother had a diagnosis of HD but had been told only women get the disease. When he began to develop suspicious symptoms he was shocked to learn that men were equally at risk.

Now, imagine a room full of patients describing their experiences with genetic testing for HD. You will discover that their expectations, fantasies, hopes, fears and personality quirks all play a role in their responses. Following are the kinds of comments you would hear.

■ ■ ■

Thirty-eight year old Betty was very nervous about requesting the test. Her anxiety skyrocketed after the blood sample was drawn and she waited 2 weeks for the result. She got no sleep at all the night before and tightly held her husband's hand in the clinic. The normal/negative test result brought tears to her eyes and she hugged her husband, hugged the genetic counselor, and hugged the doctor. She had a sense of tremendous relief and was obviously very pleased with the experience and the result.

■ ■ ■

Twenty-four-year old Linda was even more anxious about genetic testing. She was a recent college graduate and had just started a new job a pharmacist assistant. Her father had died with HD. She had ruminated about genetic testing for several years and finally decided to move forward. Linda arrived in the clinic neatly dressed in a business suit, articulate but worried. Nervously wringing her hands during counseling, she said she had finally settled on her decision to discover her genetic status. She thought the results would be most important for her career decisions, marriage plans and financial strategies. She had no physical signs of the disease and impressed our team as intelligent, careful and thoughtful. She left the clinic, got her blood drawn in the lab, and made an appointment to receive test results in four weeks. Four weeks later she failed to make her clinic appointment. When called by the counselor, she admitted that she couldn't quite bring herself to learn the results. She did, however, agree to a rescheduled visit in another four weeks. The day before the allotted time she called and canceled the appointment. She said she simply was not ready and would let us know when, and if, she changed her mind. Weeks, then months passed without hearing from her. We did not know if she had pushed the problem out of her consciousness or whether she was agonizing over the issue on a daily basis. More than a year later she called and scheduled another visit. On the appointed day, she appeared after a sleepless night with sweaty palms and a shaky voice. Her best friend was with her for support. When told the test was normal she stared straight ahead without blinking, as if she had not heard. She had to be told again, slowly and directly, "the test result is normal." She squeezed her friend's hand, sighed and shook her head in disbelief. "I was so afraid the test was positive. I don't really know what to say or do. I think I am feeling great relief, but it is going to take a while to sink in." And it probably did take a long time for her to come to grips with a new perspective on life.

■ ■ ■

Twenty-year-old Rebecca was more reserved and guarded than Betty or Linda. As an adolescent she watched her mother die with HD, and she had decided to have genetic testing as soon as she became a legal adult, at age 18. She appeared in clinic with a bit of an edge. She wore black pants with a black T-shirt, dark red lipstick, a large ring in her left ear, a small ring in her nose, short black hair with red streaks, and tattoos on both arms. Her neurological exam was entirely normal with no movements of any kind. She could not be dissuaded from the testing. When the test result was positive her subdued response was, "It figures." She seemed neither angry nor despondent, but took the news matter-of-factly. She just wanted to know the result and was ready to move on with her life. She came back to our clinic on several occasions. She found a job, had a boyfriend, and seemed to be doing reasonably well. It remains to be seen how this will play out over the coming years. Getting this information at age 18 seems a tough way to start adulthood.

■ ■ ■

Beverley's response to genetic testing was, "No way. This was terrible. Testing was the biggest mistake I ever made. My test was positive and it has ruined my life. I have been depressed and unhappy ever since and I can't stop thinking about it. If I had it to do over again I definitely would not have testing." Beverley continues to have no symptoms of HD and, taking an antidepressant, is actually functioning day-to-day without serious incidents, but she can't shake her unhappiness with the test result. She is one of those persons who was betting her test would be negative and, even after careful counseling prior to testing, was not ready to accommodate to the opposite result. She rues the day she opted to go for testing, and now she cannot put the genetic genie back in the bottle.

■ ■ ■

With curly white hair and wire-rimmed glasses, Mrs. Jacobs was 68 when she had her test. She also had no symptoms. Her mother had died with HD. Mrs. Jacobs said she was not concerned about herself, but had two children and three grandchildren and had decided to find out if they were at risk for this disease. Of course, she hoped she would be in the clear and they would have no risk. She was right that the odds were in her favor because of being asymptomatic at her age, but late onset of the disease does occasionally happen. Her test came back "abnormal" with 40 CAG repeats. She took a deep sigh and said, "Well, there you are. At least now we know. My children can decide if they want testing and I certainly hope they have escaped. I know it is possible that neither one has the gene and that is my greatest wish." Her two adult children were aware of her testing, and now the next decision was up to them. The genetic string would continue to play out in her family.

■ ■ ■

Charles played the genetic testing game very carefully. He understood that, by federal law, insurance companies cannot deny health insurance on the basis of a genetic disease or a genetic test demonstrating a genetic disease mutation. But there are no such regulations regarding life, disability or long-term care insurance. A positive genetic test could result in denial or a greatly increased premium for those three types of policies. Charles signed up for both life insurance and an expensive long-term care insurance policy prior to testing. He could honestly state he had no known genetic diseases. To his great relief his genetic test was normal and he promptly canceled the long-term care insurance, which would have been a serious financial burden for him, but a burden he was ready to accept had his test shown the HD mutation.

■ ■ ■

Robert would not be in the room to discuss genetic testing. Forty-five years old, he was from a small farming community about 150 miles away from the clinic. His father had died with HD. Robert came to the clinic with his wife. He was calm, articulate and determined to proceed with testing. His neurological exam was normal but his genetic test revealed the HD mutation. He accepted his positive result with a nod of his head and a shrug of his shoulders. He said he wasn't too surprised and was resigned to the outcome. Unfortunately, what he meant by "resignation" was unexpected. He returned home and a few days later killed himself with a shotgun. This came as a complete shock. He had given no clue to his family or to our clinic team that this was his intention. We agonized over what we might have done differently to prevent this outcome.

Why did Robert choose to kill himself after getting his genetic test result? Perhaps he had seen his father consumed by the severely debilitating final stage of HD. Perhaps Robert could not face that future for himself. The risk for suicide hovers in the background of every conversation about HD. It is an especially worrisome outcome lurking in the shadows surrounding every test for the HD mutation, an outcome every genetic counselor, physician and family member tries to avoid. Suicide represents the cause of death in about 5–6% of persons with HD—five times higher than the national average. It can happen at any time but is most common when a person at risk decides he or she is developing symptoms.

■ ■ ■

Monica should have been delighted with her test results. There was good news. She had not inherited the mutation associated with HD. But the results made Monica uneasy, even a little depressed. Her sister and brother had previously been tested and both had the HD mutation. Monica had always been very close to her siblings. Now her response was, "Why me? Why didn't I get the bad gene instead of my brother and sister? I love them so much I want them to be the lucky ones. I can handle bad news better than they can. Why do I have to watch them suffer while I escaped?" Monica had "survivor guilt." She felt the need to carry the burden for her family and let her siblings off the genetic hook. Now she felt depressed, almost embarrassed, that she was the lucky one and her brother and sister had lost the genetic roll of the dice. It would take years for her to accommodate to this new, uneasy position in her family.

■ ■ ■

Perhaps the most unusual motivation I have ever seen for requesting the HD genetic test was presented by Marvin. He was driving to work one morning, listening to the local radio station. It was a pleasant day, not raining, a cup of coffee was in the holder and traffic surprisingly light on the freeway. The newscaster related a breaking story about a woman who had just jumped off the Aurora bridge. Marvin registered it as a sad story, but certainly of no personal importance to him. He was wrong. On arriving at work a phone call informed him that the bridge jumper had been his mother. She had HD, and he had been estranged from her for many years, with essentially no contact. Now, in a dramatic and unexpected way, this episode brought him back face to face with his risk for HD. He was forced to rethink his avoidance of the topic and he decided it was time to engage this genetic reality and seek his own genetic testing. Within a few days, Marvin appeared in our clinic with this story and began the counseling and testing process. The genetic wheel of fortune was going to take another spin.

■ ■ ■

A different scenario took place when, to complete the genetic testing spectrum, Justin had this to say about his experience (printed with his permission):

> I was 18 years old when I came in for the test. I had just been accepted to college and was pretty terrified that, one day, I wouldn't be able to remember the things I was about to learn. I don't really remember a lot of the conversations beforehand or talking with the social workers. I just remember needing to know.
>
> This is why, when I came in for the second appointment, the way you gave me my result couldn't have been better. We went into the

office (my mom was there with me) and the first thing you said was "Your test came back normal, you do not have Huntington's disease."

I remember sitting there in silence for a few seconds because, of course, I had spent the day convincing myself that the test would come back positive.

I remember saying something like "Way Good," which isn't something anyone says but I might have been trying to say more than one thing at once. The full impact didn't sink in until later that day when I started calling everyone I knew to tell them the good news.

You should also know that, after that day, I felt like I had a new lease on life and I have been taking advantage of it. I am about to begin my final year of my Master's degree (I'm studying computational finance and getting my MBA), I start a new job as a risk analyst at American Investments next week, I speak 3 languages and I have traveled extensively throughout Europe, Asia, and South America. I run half-marathons and I rock climb. I say "yes" to everything. I practice yoga and brew my own beer.

I'm not telling you these things to brag. On the contrary, I'm telling you these things to say thank you. I know my genetic code was determined long before I ever met you, but the way you gave me the result and the conversation afterward has really driven me and helped me live the life I've wanted to live.

My Mom and Grandfather and Aunt have since passed away from complications resulting from Huntington's disease. My Aunt had a terrible time with HD, abused by a boyfriend and ended up malnourished and abandoned. My mom was the last to go and she passed away about 2 weeks ago. I was her only child and my Aunt didn't have any children. Everyone else who had a chance to have HD in the family has been tested and the result has come back negative.

Huntington's disease is no longer in my family.

I know you have to give bad news to people on a pretty regular basis, and I can't imagine how difficult that must be. People take a huge risk in getting that test and, after seeing what it does to your family, it can be a very scary test to take. I hope that getting some good news from someone that you gave good news to 10 years ago will brighten up your day, at least a little.

Thus, the reactions to genetic testing for HD are as varied as human nature. As healthcare providers we often try to predict a person's response. We make every effort to be as careful and as supportive as possible. We think we have a pretty good idea how most people will respond, but are sometimes very wrong and try to always be prepared for unexpected reactions. I suppose it's part of the imprecise "art" of genetic counseling, which can become incredibly complicated in surprising ways.

References

1. Genova, L. *Still Alice*. Simon & Shuster, New York, 2009.
2. Genova, L. *Inside the O'Briens*. Simon & Shuster, New York, 2015.

PART I

Interacting with the Legal and Mental Healthcare Systems

Persons with Huntington disease can be impulsive, have impaired judgment capacity, and be oblivious to the consequences of their actions. The combination of these traits can lead to serious and sometimes life-changing complications. Individuals may break the law and wind up in jail or prison, or their misbehaviors may lead to hospitalization. Difficult questions arise regardless of which course is taken, prison or hospital:

- How long should they be detained?
- How should they be treated?
- Can they be hospitalized against their will?
- What happens after their release?

- Can violence be a result of the brain disconnection associated with HD?
- Should persons with degenerative brain diseases be in prisons?
- What is the role of state mental institutions?

The following stories demonstrate how difficult it can be for persons with HD to navigate our legal and mental healthcare systems. Although most persons with HD do not experience some of the extreme difficulties about to be described, these vignettes demonstrate how problematic these experiences can become.

As noted in the Preface, HD is like the proverbial canary in the mine, the mine being our mental healthcare system. Homelessness, unexpected violence, suicide, family bankruptcy, and antisocial behavior can all occur with HD, and our society's inability to adequately address these problems is continually brought to our attention by the news media. Perhaps focusing on these issues in HD will help us address them in a larger context.

This section also describes the historical development of large mental hospitals, or asylums. Throughout the 19th and 20th centuries these institutions, for better or worse, played an outsized role in the world of HD. For many people with HD they were a safety net or a last stop in their lives. For medical, political and economic reasons their role has diminished in the last 40 years, but with proper support, they can still provide an important and helpful function in the overall care of persons with HD.

4

Can You Help Me?

When I first saw his twitches, I knew Johnny Cooper had Huntington disease. This wasn't surprising. When one decides to specialize in genetic diseases of the nervous system, one should be prepared to see persons whose brains are disconnecting in strange and unusual ways. This is the journey I began in 1974, when my colleagues and I started a neurogenetics clinic for adults at the University of Washington. The emphasis was on diagnosing, counseling and managing patients and families with hereditary diseases of the brain and nervous system. The clinical team consisted of a neurologist (the author during the time covered by this book), a board-certified genetics counselor, a nurse specializing in patients with degenerative diseases, and a social worker expert in dealing with patients with psychosocial problems. We never knew what kinds of problems we would see in the clinic from day to day. Sometimes, for example, it would be a middle-aged man who was difficult to understand because of slurred speech, which had been progressively worsening over the past five years. This was now combined with unsteady walking and hand tremor that made his handwriting illegible and caused him to spill coffee on his shirt (cerebellar ataxia). Sometimes it was a 30-year-old woman who was once an active child but was now in a wheelchair (muscular dystrophy). At other times it was a teenage boy whose deteriorating peripheral nerves caused deformities of the bones of his feet and slapping of his feet when walking, necessitating braces on his legs (hereditary neuropathy).

For reasons we never fully understood, the most common condition coming to the clinic was Huntington disease. Every week there was at least one, and more often, two or three families with HD seeking help with behavior problems, or abnormal movements, or disability certification requests, or genetic counseling. We quickly became the "go-to" clinic for HD because the patients often had no money, no resources, and were unable to obtain adequate care at private hospitals. That was why, in 1980, the following letter arrived in my office on lined tablet paper in a shaky handwritten scrawl:

April 1, 1980
#77423

Dear Dr. Bird,

Can you help me? I have the Huntington's corea (sic). My mother had it too. I am in the Walla Walla Pen. I don't feel at ease around a lot of people and break out in a sweat and start twitching and they think I'm that way all the time which I'm not. People run in the other direction when they see me coming. I can see the handwriting on the wall and had better act fast. When I get out do you have a clinic where you see people with the corea? Please let me know.

Sincerely,
Johnny Cooper
#77423

I replied with the following short letter on official University of Washington letterhead.

> *Dear Mr. Cooper,*
> *Thank you for your letter. We have a clinic at the University of Washington hospital that evaluates and follows patients with Huntington's Chorea. We would be pleased to see you in our clinic if you were living in the Seattle area. Clinic appointments can be made by calling phone number 206-444-3981.*
>
> *Sincerely,*
> *Thomas D. Bird, MD*
> *University of Washington*

Mr. Cooper's letter had been written in the Washington State prison in Walla Walla, Washington (Figure 4.1). The high, thick concrete walls of this penitentiary with guard towers perched on the corners

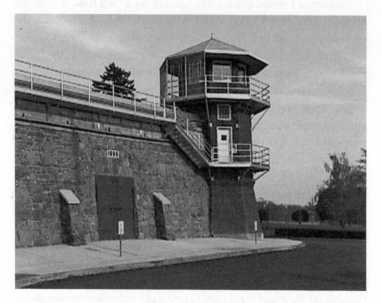

Figure 4.1 ▪ Washington State Penitentiary in Walla Walla, where Johnny Cooper with Huntington disease wrote his letter asking for help.

were reminiscent of a 19th century Army fort standing isolated on sentry duty on the Great Plains. Walla Walla ("the town so nice they named it twice") was the site of the infamous Whitman family massacre in 1847, when Native Americans became suspicious that the missionaries were infecting them with deadly measles. Now the region is best known for rolling hills of wheat and vineyards producing high-quality wines. The prison, which provides steady employment for the town, was opened in 1886 when Washington was still a territory. The remote location was undoubtedly meant to keep criminals far from the growing population west of the Cascade Mountains. Known locally as "the wall," "the hill," or "cement mama," the prison was constructed with extra-heavy bricks from a neighboring brickyard and huge rocks dragged over from the Columbia River. The dark cells and hallways were only lit with candles until electricity was introduced in 1902. Now the prison is always full, with more than 2,400 inmates who spend their time producing 2 million license plates each year. Johnny Cooper was one of those inmates.

I assumed I would not see Mr. Cooper for a long time, if ever. The state penitentiary in Walla Walla is for persons who have committed serious crimes, not petty larceny, and he was likely to be there for years. In fact, at the time Johnny Cooper was incarcerated there, the big cement mama went through a tense period of inmate murders, riots, lockdowns, lawsuits, and a wildcat strike by corrections officers.[1]

Just a few months after receiving the letter quoted here, a middle-aged man appeared in my clinic in a tattered, checkered sport coat, probably fresh from the Salvation Army. It was Johnny Cooper. He had the slightly disheveled appearance of someone who tried to be presentable but has difficulty with buttons, ties, and a razor. He had a weathered, round face with eyes that tended to look down or to the side when he was talking. Direct eye contact was not his forte. The occasional sudden, irregular jerks of his hands, shoulders, and face quickly confirmed in my mind that he did indeed have Huntington's.

I told him I was surprised to see him so soon.

"Well," he said, "Walla Walla is way overcrowded. I told them I had the chorea. They told me if I could find a place that would take care of my disease on the outside they would let me go. I showed them your letter and here I am."

I asked him why he had been in the Walla Walla Pen, and with a wry smile he said, "I stole some things," then paused and added, "more than once." He showed no interest in providing more details. There seemed to be a lot he wasn't telling me, and I didn't pry.

He related that his mother had died about 10 years earlier with HD. He was very proud of the fact that she was born on the first day of January in the year 1900, the first baby of the 20th century in her small town. This was supposed to be "lucky," but it didn't turn out that way for her. She had spent several years in Northern State Psychiatric Hospital 60 miles north of Seattle. Johnny himself had no brothers or sisters and no children. His mental abilities seemed perfectly intact and his physical examination indicated no problems other than his occasional muscle twitches. I wondered how someone with HD had survived for many years inside the prison. He didn't have much to say about it. Apparently, he quietly followed the rules and kept a low profile.

We talked about HD, its variety of symptoms and slow progression. I told him he did not require any medication at the present time and we would like to see him about twice a year. He agreed, we shook hands, and off he went.

A few months later I received a phone call from a parole officer who said he was calling about Johnny Cooper. He wanted to know if I had seen Johnny and if it was true that he had a brain disease. We chatted briefly about Johnny and his HD. He then told me he just wanted to let me know that Johnny had stolen a sweater from the local Nordstrom's. The officer had Johnny return the sweater and he did not report the infraction because he considered Johnny "a pretty good guy." He knew the Walla Walla Prison was full and he did not particularly want Johnny to go back. He asked me to please remind Johnny not to steal things.

The next time Johnny came to the clinic we talked about the sweater theft and I told him he would be in big trouble if it happened again. He said he would try not to let it happen again, but mentioned matter-of-factly that sometimes he just couldn't help himself.

The following year I had another call from the parole officer. He said, "Unfortunately, you will not be seeing Johnny Cooper again. He is back in Walla Walla."

"What happened?"

"He burglarized a home and got caught. Even worse, he made a big mistake. He hit the home of Victor Rossellini, Seattle's premier restaurateur and cousin of the former governor, Albert Rossellini. When they discovered he was out on parole, he went back to Walla Walla real fast."

Did Johnny Cooper's compulsive stealing have anything to do with his HD? I think it did, but the connection is complicated and difficult to pin down. On the one hand, compulsive behaviors, antisocial behaviors and difficulty with impulse control are well-recognized symptoms of HD. On the other hand, why stealing and why Johnny Cooper? Most people with HD are law-abiding citizens who do not steal things. The deterioration of nerve cells in persons with HD does not always follow the same pattern. Different areas of the brain relate to different behaviors in very complex ways. Johnny's disease pattern must have disrupted some brain circuitry in a special way. Furthermore, who knows what other genes and background brain systems were present in this single individual that allowed his disease to play out in the way it did. And, of course, I know nothing about the social environment surrounding his early years and how that molded and directed his behavior. These are questions and themes that occur over and over again in discussions of brain disease and mental illness, and they will reappear often in the stories that follow.

Johnny asked a perfectly good question: Could I help him? Could I help anyone with HD, and how much and in what ways could I help? What neither Johnny nor I knew at the time was that I had already started on a 40-year odyssey seeing hundreds of families with HD and constantly asking these very questions. Let me next introduce you to Brian Bachman, whose story resonates in many ways with that of Johnny.

Reference

1. Murray C. *Unusual Punishment: Inside the Walla Walla Prison, 1970–1985.* Washington State University Press, Pullman, WA, 2016.

5

It Was Awful

It was awful. I was 21. I walked into my house and found my father dead on the stairway. Can you believe it? He had taken an overdose or had a heart attack and collapsed on the stairs. I didn't like him. He was mean and nasty to me. But he WAS my FATHER! And then the next week my mother died. She had liver failure. She was alcoholic. Their funerals were the same weekend. It was awful. I didn't know my mother's family. They were from back east. Some relative, a cousin or somebody, showed up at her funeral and said, "Oh, by the way, her family has Huntington's chorea. We think her father had it." I had never heard of Huntington's chorea. I did a little reading about it. It was awful. I was only 21. I mostly forgot about it, but that's why I'm here today. I'm worried I might have it.

■ ■ ■

That was the story of Brian Bachman. He appeared in our clinic in his late 40s. He was agitated when telling his story, then would calm down, but was clearly and deeply concerned about his situation. You could hear the urgent sadness in his voice. He was a tall, athletically built man with wavy hair, gray at the temples, square jaw and deep-set dark eyes. He clearly had been a handsome young man, but now had a bit too much weight loss and a sad, forlorn facial appearance suggesting a stressful life. His teeth were cigarette stained and in need of repair. He was intelligent and thoughtful, but his conversation was rambling and disjointed.

When asked about other family members he said, "I had two brothers. My youngest brother died in his 20s of alcohol and drug abuse. He was a mess. My other brother is still alive. We're not in close contact. We didn't get along. I think he is seen at the VA hospital. He's had drug problems, too. He may have the Huntington's."

I was stunned by his story. It was a déjà vu experience for me. I had not recognized this initially, but now realized I knew the Bachman family. In fact, I knew them from 25 or 30 years before.

Back when I had been a neurology resident in training, we had a 16-year-old teenage boy admitted to our hospital neurology service who was in a coma from a drug overdose. We thought it was odd that he had no visitors. One day, his father suddenly appeared. He was ultra-clean-cut, wearing a full gray suit and dark red necktie. He first briefly visited his son, but then took me aside and said he had something important to tell me. His message was, "I don't want our family name in the newspapers or on TV. This is important. This is private. Keep it private." His tone was threatening. I assured him it would all stay private. As an afterthought he asked, "Will he recover?" I indicated that, yes, his condition was stable, he was improving and he should recover completely. The father said nothing, but left the hospital abruptly. I distinctly remember the family name was Bachman. This is because the father was wealthy and owned a local construction company. For many years thereafter I would occasionally see trucks in Seattle with "Bachman Construction" on the side panel. I now realized that this was Brian's father. And the boy with the drug overdose was Brian's younger brother, who apparently died 10 or 12 years after that overdose, from alcohol and drug abuse. Furthermore, I realized I had seen Brian's other brother at the VA hospital. He did, indeed, have a diagnosis of HD. He had never told me about his two brothers. It was startling to have this distraught family reappear in a completely different context more than 25 years later.

Meanwhile, as these memories were running through my mind, Brian continued his story. He had left Seattle soon after his parents' funerals, wandered the country, and eventually ended up in New York City. His natural good looks resulted in some photography gigs. One thing led to another and he soon became a highly successful male fashion model. He jet-setted between New York, Paris and Milan. "Look," he said, "Here is my portfolio." He pulled a large, thick envelope from his backpack. Emptying the envelope on the table, he spread out dozens of old photographs. Several were torn and many were folded at the corners and yellow around the edges. But there, unmistakably, was Brian in a tuxedo standing next to a blonde in a blue ballgown, both of them admiring a jet black Rolls Royce. And there was Brian in an open-collar pink dress shirt and a tweed sports coat, smoking a cigarette and extolling the virtues of Benson and Hedges. Another had him modeling a line of men's suits, and in yet another, Brian was in swimming trunks sitting by a pool with his well-tanned, muscular body. There were also several color and black-and-white headshots of Brian taken from various angles and in a variety of lighting. In his favorite romantic shot he was about to kiss a girl, for the cover of *Esquire* (Figure 5.1). He was only 22 years old, but had already made it to the cover of a national magazine.

Needless to say, this was not our usual clinic patient, and we were all duly impressed. Brian went on to say that he made pretty good money, but spent it all as fast as he made it. The fashion modeling business only lasts so long, and age, cigarettes and alcohol took their toll. He returned to Seattle, was briefly married, had a child, and then divorced. He had been unemployed for years. He now had no money and lived in a cheap one-room apartment. His nutrition was marginal. He used to be a good tennis player and still played the game. However, he said his coordination was lousy and his memory and concentration were no longer any good. He had begun thinking about the Huntington's in his mother's family, had read about genetic testing, and wanted to find out if he had inherited the disease.

We spent considerable time discussing HD with Brian and the pros and cons of genetic testing. He grasped all the key factors and felt strongly that he wanted the test. It was not clear whether he had signs of the disease. On the one hand, he had nothing that could be called true involuntary movements. On the other hand, his coordination was a bit

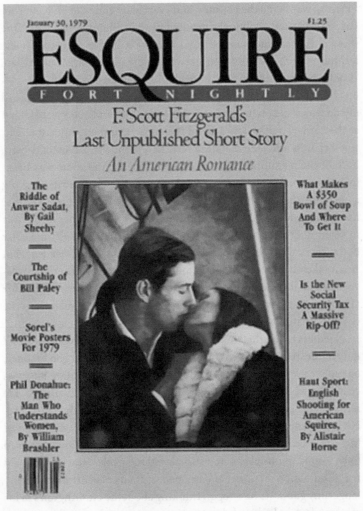

Figure 5.1 ■ At age 22, Brian Bachman, just beginning his career as a model, appeared on the cover of *Esquire*. (With permission of Brian, photographer Dan Weaks, and *Esquire*.)

off and something was not quite right about his thinking. His memory was excellent but his conversation was rambling, tangential, and it was difficult to bring his focus back to the topic at hand. He returned in a few weeks and his test result was positive. He had inherited the mutation for HD. He said he was not surprised by the results, and he was not going to change his lifestyle. He indicated he planned to give the genetic news to his ex-wife and his now young-adult daughter.

The saga of Brian and his family did not stop there. We continued to see Brian about every six months, but we also began to interact with his brother, Carl.

Brian's brother Carl was being followed for his HD in the neurology clinic at the VA Medical Center and in Psychiatry for his alcohol and drug history and a personality disorder. He, too, was divorced with one young-adult child. Also, like Brian, he had no involuntary movements, but his judgment and personality were impaired. He had been in the Army during the Vietnam era and had several scrapes with the Military Police. After discharge he had been a carpenter for several years, but now was unemployed. He was renting a one-room basement apartment in an old house on Capitol Hill and kept in contact with his daughter. A recurrent problem was that he would disappear and his landlord and daughter would become concerned about his safety. Once he was gone for several days, and a missing persons report was filed with the police. He was eventually located sleeping in his car near a beach on the Oregon coast. He said he just liked to "get away" every once in a while.

Carl's condition slowly deteriorated over several years. He developed a few jerky movements of his face and shoulders, but nothing serious. He became more withdrawn and hyper-religious. His conversations always veered toward the Bible, and his friends and family grew tired of his religious rhetoric. Also, he became paranoid and covered his windows with aluminum foil to prevent people from watching him. His psychiatrists tried several different medications, but nothing had much effect on his behavior.

Once again, Carl disappeared for days, and his empty automobile was found parked at a lonely trailhead up in the Cascade Mountains. Carl could not be found. Several weeks later his body was discovered in a nearby river beneath an area where the trail made a sharp turn close to a steep cliff. It could never be determined whether he jumped or fell.

Carl's memorial service was an uplifting celebration of his life. I discovered that he had been active in a prison ministry. His thoughtful counseling was described as very beneficial to many of the prisoners. His brother Brian spoke at the service. Not surprisingly, his comments rambled on far longer than any of the others. But Brian had some good memories of Carl, and he was able to express the positive parts of their past relationship.

Sadly, I was reminded of a similar memorial service I had attended the previous year. Another man with more advanced HD drove into the mountains by himself and his body was also found floating in a river. He had been told that it had become impossible to care for him at home, and he was going to be admitted to the same nursing home where his father had died with HD many years before. Although it seemed likely he had decided to jump rather than go into that nursing home, there remained a possibility that he could have fallen. For that reason, I think he was able to have a full memorial service at his Catholic church. Family, friends and the priest were very kind and thoughtful in the celebration of his life.

Brian seemed to deteriorate psychologically after Carl's death. He became more depressed, withdrawn and less social. It was hard to keep him on his medications. One time the pharmacy refused to mail his meds and he refused to pick them up. I didn't want our nurse or social worker going alone to his sketchy neighborhood, so I delivered his medicines myself. It was both instructive and disappointing to see his living environment. He was in a one-bedroom flat at the end of a small, rundown apartment building. It was a sunny day, and it took a few minutes for my eyes to adjust to the darkness inside his living room. The shades were drawn and there was just a small, dim table lamp with its shade askew. Off to the side was a sofa partially covered with a ripped blanket and the pillows were on the floor. There was no TV, but a radio was tuned to a pop music station. In the back of the room a small kitchen area had a sink full of dirty dishes and a narrow table with two small wooden chairs. One wall had a rock-music poster and the other wall had a large white cloth covered with black and red Chinese characters. The room smelled of either incense or pot (or probably both).

Brian was in dirty blue jeans, bare feet and an old T-shirt. However, he said things were fine, and his only complaint was chronic insomnia. He showed me his medicine bottles. I was pleased to see that they were appropriately nearly empty and he had not been hoarding. We chatted about his health and general welfare, as well as his favorite baseball team, the Mariners. I told him that we wanted to continue to see him in the clinic, but we both knew that would be a transportation problem since he had no car, no friends with a car, and he refused to take the city bus. The county Access shuttle bus for disabled persons refused to serve him because he was considered fully ambulatory and should be able to find his own way on a Metro bus. Actually, his gait had been deteriorating, he had had several falls, and could not manage the bus system. Nevertheless, we were not able to change his transportation to Access.

Several months passed, and then our clinic nurse received a large envelope from Brian. It contained all his portfolio photographs from when he had been a fashion model. Attached was a rambling letter that basically said that he would not be needing these anymore because he had decided to "give up and throw in the towel"—obviously, a very bad sign. Already with chronic depression, it was clear that we needed to get Brian to the hospital and find a bed for him. He would not be an appropriate admission to the Neurology Service because, although he clearly had a neurological illness, he needed a locked ward and intensive psychiatric monitoring. At first, the psychiatrists were reluctant to take him. One of the arguments was that he had a "brain" disease, not a "mental" disease. The ensuing philosophical discussion about the "mind/body" problem still happens in today's medical world. I made the point that schizophrenia is also a brain disease. Bipolar disorder is a brain disease. Psychiatric diseases are brain diseases because mental activity and, therefore, mental illness originates in the brain. Having resolved the philosophical argument for the moment, we still needed to find him a bed. If he voluntarily consented to admission, that would get us over one hurdle. If he did not consent, we could still make a strong argument that he was a danger to himself. At the moment, all beds on the Psychiatry inpatient service were full, but a discharge was expected later in the day. I was able to contact Brian by phone, and he agreed to come to the hospital by taxi if we paid for it.

Brian was very reluctant to be admitted to the hospital, but I think deep down he recognized that we were his only support and we had his best interests at heart. The social worker, the nurse, and I walked him across the street to the emergency department (ED). He was placed in a small, windowless, nearly claustrophobic room furnished with a portable bed and a single chair. The emergency room boarding process had begun.

Over a period of several hours, Brian was interviewed by the ED nurse, the ED social worker, and the Psychiatry consultant. He began his conversation with each visitor by retelling the awful story of finding his father dead on the stairs, followed quickly by his mother's death and the two funerals. He never tired of telling this story and there is no question that it weighed heavily on his mind for the rest of his life. This tale had become a memory tape he would play over and over at a moment's notice. Unfortunately, the other patient who occupied a psychiatry bed was not discharged, and there continued to be no opening in the hospital. Brian spent the rest of the day and all night in the same little ED room. He also spent all the following day in the ED. Our clinic nurse brought him trays of food from the hospital cafeteria and engaged him in conversation, trying to keep his mind off his depressing circumstances. Finally, in the evening of the second day, a bed on the Psychiatry unit was vacated and Brian was admitted. This had been a frustrating experience in "ED boarding," and we were lucky Brian hadn't decompensated and bolted. It would have been an isolating and claustrophobic experience for anyone and nearly unbearable for someone fighting depression. The frequent visits from our nurse and social worker kept Brian from emotionally falling apart.

Besides treating his depression, another major goal of this admission was to leverage him out of his dreary, ramshackle apartment (which was clearly adding to his depression) and get him into an adult care home or some kind of rehab center. His depression seemed to at least partially improve on a medication change, talk therapy, and a much nicer living environment. His housing change proved to be more difficult. Adult family homes have to be paid for, and Brian had no financial resources. Apparently he would be eligible for some modest resources at age 60 but he was presently only 59. He had to be interviewed by a healthcare professional to determine if he qualified for financial assistance for an adult family home. The interview would be with Brian alone and not with any of the members of his medical and psychiatric care team. He flunked the interview and was declared ineligible for any resources. He flunked because he told the interviewer he could do everything for himself. He stated he could take the bus, shop by himself, prepare his own meals, and bathe and shower. The problem, of course, was that he couldn't do any of those things. On his occasional shopping trips he bought mostly peanut butter and cookies. He did no cooking whatsoever in his apartment. He never took the bus, and his bathing hygiene was atrocious. But none of that factual information counted. All that counted was what he said he could do. After a two-week stay, he was discharged back to his apartment. No one thought this process was headed in the right direction.

It didn't take long for things to fall apart. On his second follow-up visit a few months later, Brian was again seriously depressed. He seemed desperate, but with perfect lucidity said, "I want death with dignity. I am just asking for death with dignity." He meant this both figuratively and literally. He was referring to the relatively new Washington state law called "Death with Dignity." It is very similar to a law passed several years ago in Oregon. In this state, the program is also known as a form of physician-assisted suicide. Physicians are allowed to write a prescription for a fatal dose of barbiturate for a person seeking to end his or her life. It most commonly is used by patients with end-stage cancer or ALS (Lou Gehrig's disease). Whatever one's opinion of this law, it is not an option for persons with HD. This is because, first, the physician must declare that the patient has a fatal disease from which he or she will die in less than six months. Second, the patient cannot be depressed and must be cognitively intact. A patient with end-stage HD within six months of death (however that might be determined) is essentially never going to be cognitively intact. When this was explained to Brian, it just made him more depressed: "I just want to end it all. I just can't go on."

Clearly, it was time for another hospital admission. We explained to Brian that the goal was to make him feel better, improve his life, and get him out of that dungeon of an apartment. We knew that Brian was basically a sociable guy. Getting him into a better social environment, having him interact with other friendly people, and having clean sheets and three square meals a day was very likely to have a positive result. Fortunately, he said, "I am willing to give it a try." That meant his admission would be voluntary, and we would not have to prove he was a danger to himself or others.

We walked Brian over to the ED. The psychiatry team remembered him very well and was willing to readmit him. Of course there was no open bed, but once again a discharge was "pending." So Brian spent the rest of the day, the night and the next morning in a tiny, windowless room in the ED, his home away from home. He was back on the psychiatry floor the next afternoon.

It wasn't easy, but some things went better for Brian this time around. Everyone on his healthcare team was committed to keeping him in the hospital until he could be transferred to a better environment. He was not going to be discharged back to his unkempt apartment. In addition, Brian had recognized his deterioration over the last few months and realized he could no longer care for himself. So when a new healthcare specialist came around again to interview him, he passed the survey. He admitted that there were a lot of things he could no longer do. That was the good news. The bad news was that he just barely passed the survey and only qualified for a reimbursement of $57 per day. Not good. No adult care home was going to accept someone with such meager resources.

But the search for a new home had begun. Week after week, Brian's situation was reviewed by supervisors of numerous potential new living places. He was always rejected. However, things were actually taking a turn for the better. Brian's nutrition improved, and he gained weight. He shaved. He showered. He was active in group therapy. He was feeling better. He also turned 60 and a few more resources became available. Sure enough, a kind young woman operating an adult family home bonded with Brian. She smiled and said, "I will take him," and she did. It was almost as if she had found a friendly stray cat to adopt and nurture. After a two-month hospital stay, Brian was discharged to his new home. Great relief. High-fives all around.

At first things went well for Brian, but he was not quite out of the HD woods. After a few weeks we got word that Brian had aspirated food, gotten severe pneumonia, and had been admitted to the local hospital. In fact, the pneumonia was so bad he was admitted to their intensive care unit (ICU) and had to have a chest tube placed for drainage. This was very ominous. We all thought he was on the way out. His condition sounded terminal.

But no, Brian didn't quit. He slowly turned the corner and was moved out of the ICU. Over a period of weeks, he completely recovered and was sent back to his adult care home.

When we last saw Brian in the clinic he was a new man. His gait was unsteady, his speech was slurred, and he had a few twitches. But he was upbeat and happy. He said his life was the best it had been in years. He liked the food, he liked the atmosphere, and his liked his care provider. He gave smiles and hugs to everyone. His caretaker said that Brian had told her his awful story of finding both parents dead, the two funerals and his brothers' demise. She said that his story made her very sad and also motivated her to give him the best of care.

Not surprisingly, Brian continued to have ups and downs. He was allowed to do grocery shopping at the local Safeway for a few small items. One day, while on one of these brief shopping excursions, we received a call that he had been arrested and was in jail. He had stuffed some small packages of cookies and candies into his coat, walked out of the store, and this was noticed by a cashier. She called the police. He was quickly found with the contraband and taken to jail. He may have argued with the officer and probably appeared intoxicated (although he was not). Fortunately, we were able to arrange for his caretaker to bring his medications to the jail and he was allowed to take them. We were able to explain his situation and his disease to a kindly public defender who got the charges dropped. He was released after three days. Yes, he spent three days in jail for shoplifting a bag of cookies. Brian was unable to explain the theft other than shrug his shoulders about the temptation and his sweet tooth. This seemed to be yet another example of "disinhibited" behavior with HD, a recurring problem for many individuals. He was unable to inhibit a socially unacceptable impulse.

Brian's never-ending troubles had led to hospitals and jail, but he was never committed to a state mental institution. However, for a variety of reasons, many persons with HD are unable to survive in their communities and they spend months or years in large mental hospitals. These asylums have played an important and complex role in the history of HD. The next chapter explores how the role of those institutions has played out in the lives of several persons with HD who suffered a variety of serious mental collapses.

6

The Asylum

The embarrassment of confinement to a mental institution is one of the reasons persons with Huntington disease and similar diseases were literally hidden from view and often never mentioned again. They sometimes "disappeared" from their families. It is also one of the reasons HD initially fell behind in the world of medical research. It is not known exactly how many HD patients were committed to these psychiatric hospitals over the years, but nationally it was certainly in the thousands. Because these often seemingly menacing facilities have played such a dominant role in the history of HD, it is important to understand the development of what once were called "insane asylums."

HISTORICAL BACKGROUND OF "INSANE ASYLUMS"

In the 18th century, William Tuke, a Quaker in England, and Phillipe Pinel in France advocated fresh air, meaningful labor and compassionate care for the "insane" at a time when those persons with mental illness were shunned by society and miserably treated in prison-like institutions. Tuke attempted to develop "moral treatment" of the "insane" based on comfort care and kindness rather than control, isolation and punishment. In the 19th century, following Tuke's lead, James Crichton Browne became superintendent of an institution in West Yorkshire with the intimidating name of the West Riding Pauper Lunatic Asylum. Applying Tuke's and Pinel's ideas, this facility successfully incorporated, at least for a while, the improvements they had championed. Later in the late 19th century, Dorothea Dix took up this theme in the United States where many states, including my home state of Washington, were trying to follow this more compassionate model.

Washington was a relatively new state, having been admitted to the Union as the 42nd state, in 1889. One of the earliest settlements was Fort Steilacoom, near the heavily forested southern end of Puget Sound. It was there that Native Americans traded valuable beaver pelts for blankets and cookware. Ulysses Grant probably wandered through the fort early in his career. In 1871 the population of the territory was large enough that a place was required to house mentally disturbed citizens. Initially, 21 persons were given asylum in the now-unused fort. Following the Alaska gold rush there was an economic boom in Western Washington. The state legislature provided funds for a new asylum on the old military grounds. The new building opened in 1889, the same year Washington became a state, and just over 3 years after the opening of the prison in Walla Walla. The territory (and then the state) was simultaneously trying to remove from circulation in general society both criminals and the mentally insane. Over the ensuing decades the facility grew dramatically, adding both buildings and patients. The institution became known as Western State Hospital (WSH), or just "Western." By the 1930s and 1940s, the patient census was always well over 2,000 and reached more than

3,000 in the 1950s, including many patients with HD. There were no really good treatments for serious psychiatric disease, and it was not unusual for patients to spend years, decades or even the rest of their lives at Western. For several decades, Western had its own farm across the road from the main hospital that included a dairy, where patients provided most of the labor. Hard work and sunshine were considered highly therapeutic. The farm also generated income for the hospital.

Washington was not alone in trying to deal with its mentally ill population. In 1883, just 6 years prior to the opening of WSH, the state of Oregon established its "insane asylum" in the capital city of Salem. This Oregon State Mental Hospital has a long and controversial history. It was featured in Ken Kesey's novel, *One Flew Over the Cuckoo's Nest*, and subsequently was turned into a Hollywood icon in 1975 by Jack Nicholson.

The eastern part of the Unites States, with its huge population, was also building mental institutions. One of the largest of these asylums in the country was Creedmoor Hospital, in Queens, New York (Figure 6.1). Woody Guthrie, the American folk singer who wrote "This Land Is Your Land" and was the nation's most famous personality with HD, was hospitalized and died there in the 1960s (Figure 6.2). In 1959 Creedmoor had an enormous population of 7,000 patients. This was literally a city within a city and probably far too large to be adequately maintained or controlled. Over the years, undoubtedly large numbers of patients with HD passed through its doors, never to leave.

TREATMENT IN THE ASYLUM

Asylum means "shelter, refuge or sanctuary," which it was, but treatment could be problematic. In 1937 there were approximately 450,000 patients in 417 asylums in the United States. The diseases being treated included general paresis of the insane (also called GPS, a brain form of tertiary syphilis), schizophrenia, Huntington's chorea, shell shock in veterans of World War I, melancholia (depression), and senile and presenile dementia, which we now know to be usually Alzheimer disease. Treatments were generally ineffective and limited to locked wards, straitjackets, cold-water shock, and farm work. There were no

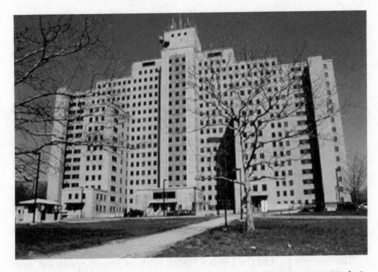

Figure 6.1 ■ Creedmoor Psychiatric Hospital in Queens, New York. In 1959 it had a population of 7,000 patients. Woody Guthrie spent the last year of his life here.

effective medicines, although bromides or phenobarbital were often used. Later came the dangerous insulin shock therapy, which was occasionally fatal and then no longer used, followed in the 1930s and 40s by electroshock (electroconvulsive therapy—ECT), which is still in use today.

For about a decade between the mid-1940s and mid-1950s, WSH performed frontal lobotomies. Dr. Walter Freemen, the physician who popularized the procedure, spent a brief time at Western. Freeman got the idea of frontal lobotomy from a Portuguese neuropsychiatrist, Egas Moniz, who first suggested the procedure in the 1930s. The simple concept was that the surgery would disconnect the source of abnormal behavior in the frontal lobes from the rest of the brain. This was initially considered a medical breakthrough in the treatment of mental illness, and Moniz received the Nobel Prize in 1949. Freeman perfected some of his techniques, on patients at St. Elizabeth's Hospital, a large asylum in Washington, DC. At first, a frontal lobotomy was a major operation performed by a neurosurgeon in a hospital operating room. In order to

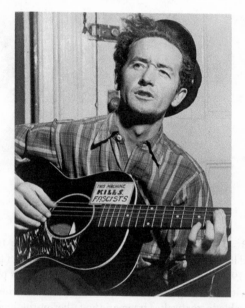

Figure 6.2 ◼ Woody Guthrie, who in 1941 wrote folk songs about building dams on the Columbia River in Washington State, died at age 55 in 1967 at Creedmore Hospital in New York.

greatly reduce the cost and make the procedure more readily available, Dr. Freeman developed a technique which he called a "transorbital leucotomy" (Figure 6.3). This was an outpatient procedure that he said could be performed by a quickly trained psychiatrist or neurologist. Instead of anesthesia, the patient was briefly stunned to unconsciousness with electroshock. The procedure was then performed with a thin knife blade or "pick" inserted under the eyelid, poked through the thin bone at the top of the eye socket and into the frontal lobe. This was done rapidly on both sides; the whole procedure took less than an hour. Dr. Freeman actually drove around the country in a vehicle he termed the "lobotomobile" demonstrating the procedure in a wide variety of hospitals and institutions. It is estimated that 50,000 lobotomies were performed in this country between 1938 and 1955, including the sisters of John F. Kennedy and Tennessee Williams, coincidentally both named Rose. In fact, in 1950 alone about 5,000 lobotomies were

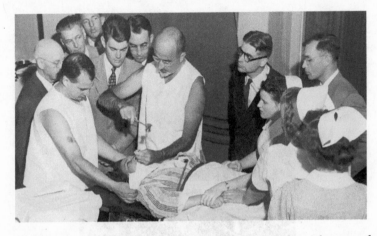

Figure 6.3 ■ Dr. Walter Freeman demonstrating the technique of transorbital lobotomy to a group of attentive doctors, students and nurses in the late 1940s. His textbook describes performing this procedure on a patient with Huntington disease (from https://www.themedicalbag.com/despicabledoctor/walter-freeman-the-father-of-the-lobotomy).

performed in the United States. At that time, Western's most famous patient was Frances Farmer. A talented Seattle-born Hollywood actress, she was perhaps most famous for her dual role in the Academy Award–winning 1936 film *Come and Get It*. It is apparently well established that she had electroconvulsive treatments at Western, but the rumor has never been substantiated that she also had a lobotomy.

Since persons with HD were often institutionalized and lobotomies were common, it is likely that many of these operations were performed on patients with HD. I was looking for proof that a lobotomy had actually been done on someone with HD. It was not easy to document, but I finally found the evidence. Careful inspection of the two books written on lobotomy, by Freeman and Watts, reveal that their Case #342 had HD.[1] The description of this patient is brief and terse. It is simply noted that his involuntary movements were not improved by the lobotomy but he was "relieved" of disturbing obsessive preoccupations. Undoubtedly, many more HD "cases" (perhaps more than 100) also had lobotomies in the other 400 asylums.

Freeman's initial neurosurgical colleague withdrew from the partner-ship because he thought transorbital lobotomies were too cavalier and should not have replaced the more major procedure performed in the operating room by a trained surgeon.

In the middle to late decades of the 20th century (1940–1990), on any given day, WSH typically had a dozen patients with HD, once having a census of 20 cases of HD in the 1970s. During much of this time Western had its own neurologist. I spoke with him on many occasions and saw numerous copies of his clinical notes. He was a committed eugenicist. He thought all persons with HD should be sterilized and advised all family members at risk to never have chil-dren. He considered this the only way to eliminate the "scourge" of HD from society. Many physicians agreed with him, and the families felt rejected and shamed.

DEINSTITUTIONALIZATION

As in all psychiatric hospitals throughout the country, things changed dramatically for WSH in the 1960s. Antipsychotic medications had been developed and introduced into clinical practice. These medications greatly improved symptoms and behavior in vast num-bers of patients with severe psychiatric disorders such as schizo-phrenia, bipolar disease and depression. In the 1970s and '80s there was a major reduction in the populations of state psychiatric hospitals. Patients were discharged in droves, with the anticipated strategy of following them as outpatients while maintaining them on their medications. This "deinstitutionalization" had started before the dis-covery of antipsychotic drugs, but was accelerated by the advent of these medications. Many hospitals were closed, including Northern State Hospital, the other psychiatric institution in the western portion of Washington. This happened soon after Johnny Cooper's mother (whom we met in Chapter 4) died there. Unfortunately, this new out-patient strategy frequently didn't work. Patients stopped taking their medication and then disappeared from the clinic rolls. Also, the state and federal governments were so pleased with saving money on the closure of institutions that they failed to adequately fund the outpatient programs.

This sad history of the failure to anticipate the volume and complexity of care required by thousands of patients with mental illness is expertly described by E. Fuller Torrey, in his book *American Psychosis*. He summarizes the rejection of state hospitals by the Federal Interagency Committee on Mental Health in 1962, noting that this rejection

> would have profound effects on the subsequent failure of the emerging system. Because no Committee member really understood what the hospitals were doing, there was nobody who could explain to the committee that large numbers of the patients had a brain impairment that precluded their understanding of their illness and need for medication; and that a small number of the patients had a history of dangerousness and required confinement and treatment. Nobody could explain to the committee that the state hospitals were playing a role in protecting the public, and in protecting mentally ill individuals from being victimized or becoming homeless. Whatever their other shortcomings, state mental health hospitals were still functioning as asylums in the original sense of the term.[2]

Western State Hospital is still suffering from this deinstitutionalization. Now in the 21st century, it is frequently in the news, and the news is not usually good.[3-5] The hospital has been under a persistent threat of losing federal funding (which would be a disaster) because of a variety of procedural and care-delivery deficiencies. Several high-profile and potentially dangerous patients have escaped, and eventually returned. Workers have been injured by patients, patients have been injured by workers, and several hundred employee positions remain unfilled. Waiting times for admission are too long. Disturbed citizens desperately needing care cannot get in, and the hospital director has said she would go to jail, if necessary, to highlight the broken system.[6] An improved environment and better resources are badly needed.

THE MORGUE AT WESTERN STATE HOSPITAL

My most memorable trip to Western was many years ago, on a remarkable journey to collect a brain. It should come as no surprise that research on human diseases of the brain requires dissection of the actual brains after death, followed by microscopic, biochemical and molecular analysis of the tissue. The brain must be carefully removed from the skull through the process of a brain autopsy, conducted by a neuropathologist. My friend and colleague, Dr. Mark Sumi, is a superb neuropathologist who has those exact talents.

We had been studying neurochemical changes in brains of patients with HD, and in addition to normal control tissue we needed brain tissue from patients with some other similar degenerative neurological disease. Early-onset familial Alzheimer disease (AD) perfectly fit this category. It was genetic, onset of symptoms was often in the 40s, and there was a severe, progressive decline over about 10 years.

I had been evaluating and following just such a family with early-onset familial AD. One February night, I received a call from the front-desk telephone operator at WSH. A 49-year-old woman with advanced dementia in this family was a patient there, and the operator had been instructed to notify me when she died. The operator knew my role was to obtain the woman's brain and that all the proper consent forms had been signed by the family. She said the body was being moved to the hospital morgue as we spoke. I called Mark Sumi, who had agreed to assist me on this project, and off we went. We stopped by the medical school in Seattle and picked up a two-gallon plastic container with ice and another with the chemical preservative formalin. It was late at night as we headed south to Steilacoom. Naturally, it was raining, but it was much worse than the usual light rain. It was a thunderstorm with all the lightening pyrotechnics. We pulled into the desolate grounds of Western, and the old brick buildings had a dark, brooding aura that was only intensified by the storm. The operator gave me the keys to the morgue building, which she indicated was around in back of the main hospital. The hospital policeman would show us the way. We followed the policeman in his patrol car around the corner. He stopped, pointed

his finger straight ahead, and clearly had no intention of going further.
I suspect he knew our purpose. His headlights shown on a small, old,
brick building surrounded by untrimmed bushes and overgrown grass
(Figure 6.4). The building sat unused because no autopsies had been
done at Western for many years. Dr. Sumi and I unlocked the door,
stepped inside, and found the light switch. The building contained just
a single musty room with cabinets off to the side and one ceiling light
with a metal shade. In the center of the room was a large steel table, on
top of which was a body covered with a sheet.

We confirmed identification of the body with a name tag tied to her
big toe. It is always an odd feeling when participating in the autopsy

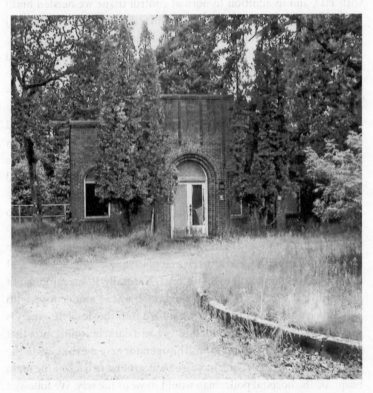

Figure 6.4 ■ Autopsy morgue at Western State Hospital, unused for
many years and destroyed in 2011, making way for new construction.
(Photo provided courtesy of Mathew Rumbaugh.)

of someone you knew as a patient. This woman experienced mild memory loss in her late 30s and her husband had brought her to our clinic because of her strong family history of dementia. There was no doubt she was developing the family disease. I recall she was not concerned about herself, but was very sad to realize her two young children were now at risk for the same condition. When she reached age 47, her husband could no longer care for her at home and they had no financial resources. Her life ended at WSH, since her husband had requested a brain autopsy to be used for research, in the hope of advancing knowledge about her disease; this is what brought us to the morgue on such dreary February night. The body under the sheet was the young woman I had met 10 years before.

Dr. Sumi found appropriate tools of his trade in the cabinets, including knives, scalpels, scissors and thin surgical gloves. I will not give all the details, but the rain bouncing off the roof and windows accompanied by occasional thunder and lightning produced an eerie theatrical effect that I will never forget. The turning back of the scalp with a scalpel was essentially bloodless. Dr. Sumi complained about the small electric saw he used to remove the top of the skull because it was dull and apparently had not been operated for a very long time. The brain was deftly removed from the base of the skull, and with scissors Dr. Sumi cut away the thick, fibrous, pale white dura that covered and protected the brain. Holding the brain carefully in both hands as if presenting a gift, it was readily apparent that it was smaller than expected and showed diffuse atrophy (shrinkage). The light brown brain tissue was visible in between the myriad rivulets of blue blood vessels covering the organ like the venous pattern on the back of your hand. Placing the brain on the end of the steel tabletop, Dr. Sumi divided it into right and left halves with a long, sharp autopsy blade reminiscent of a bread knife. Half the brain went into the container of formalin for future microscopic analysis and the other half was put on ice for biochemical testing. We draped the sheet back over her body, doused the light, and locked the door. I returned the keys to the operator with a thank you and noted that the policeman had disappeared. On the freeway heading back to Seattle through the fog and downpour, Dr. Sumi remarked that he was driving especially carefully. With a laugh he quipped that he would not want to get in an accident and have to explain to a police officer why we had two half human brains in the trunk. Certainly this was a night to remember, an association with WSH that will never be erased from my memory. The brain tissue we collected that night turned out to be very valuable. It contributed to the eventual genetic identification of the brain disease in that woman's family, a rare form of inherited AD that is similar in many ways to HD.

Brain removal for research purposes is highly relevant to HD. Actual brain tissue from persons with HD is necessary for neuroscientists to unravel at the cellular and chemical levels what is actually happening in the nerve cells and their connections. It remains poorly understood how the mutant protein produced by the abnormal HD gene causes degeneration of neurons. A better understanding of these mechanisms could provide important clues to the design of successful treatments, and brain tissue is needed to advance this research.

To carry forward the asylum theme, in the next chapter we will visit Western State Hospital and meet several patients with HD who, for a variety of reasons, were committed to that institution.

References

1. Freeman W, Watts JW. *Psychosurgery: In the Treatment of Mental Disorders and Intractable Pain*, 2nd ed. Charles C. Thomas, Springfield, IL, 1950, p. 349.
2. Torrey, EF. *American Psychosis*. Oxford University Press, New York, 2014, p. 45.
3. Bellisle M. Washington in trouble again for mental health services; judge issues fine. *Seattle Times*, July 20, 2016.
4. Seattle Times Editorial Board. Patients in limbo: where's the urgency for fixes at Western State Hospital? *Seattle Times*, July 2, 2016.
5. O'Sullivan J. Official stands by order to fix Western psychiatric hospital woes. *Seattle Times*, August 3, 2016.
6. O'Sullivan J. Western State Hospital CEO ordered to jail for keeping dementia patient on waitlist. *Seattle Times*, June 10, 2016.

7

Meeting Huntington Disease Patients at Western State

I n the 1980s I was asked to consult on several persons with Huntington disease at Western State Hospital (WSH) and provide a seminar on the disease to the staff. As noted in the previous chapter, Western is the large, state-funded, inpatient psychiatric hospital for the western, most populous half of Washington. I readily agreed and the following week, along with our clinic nurse, social worker and genetic counselor, we were off on a field trip to Western. The hospital is sited in Steilacoom, a suburb of Tacoma, about an hour drive from our clinic. We arrived at the hospital in late morning. The large, brick buildings were old and somewhat intimidating, but at least not looming out of the midnight hour of a gothic novel (Figure 7.1). The main administration

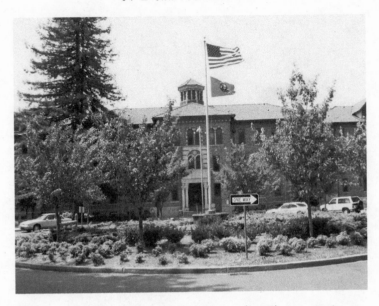

Figure 7.1 ■ Western State Hospital (WSH) in Steilacoom, Washington. This psychiatric hospital had a population of more than 3,000 patients in the 1950s and has been "home" to hundreds of patients with HD.

building was topped by a large cupola, apparently a Victorian architectural touch, but oddly reminiscent of a guard tower.

Our interactions with the staff were rewarding. The nurses, social workers and physicians were clearly dedicated and committed to the best care. They were acquainted with the details of their patients and eager to learn all we could tell them about HD.

Following an in-service seminar we walked to the neurology ward, negotiating a series of vacant hallways with multiple locked doors. It felt like walking through an intricate puzzle box with one drawer leading to another, then another, then another. The halls had no furniture or wall art of any kind. We entered the locked neurology unit, which had approximately 20 patients with a variety of brain problems. The large day room was clean and light, but sparsely furnished with a few metal tables and a variety of straight-backed wooden chairs and two old stuffed easy chairs. The walls were painted pale hospital green.

The windows were tall and the ceilings were high, reflecting the age of the building. Without carpeting, the occasional loud voice would echo around the room. There were patients with brain trauma, "burned out" encephalitis, strokes, Alzheimer and other dementias. The common theme was people with severe behavioral problems that could not be adequately managed elsewhere. The patients had failed attempts at care in a variety of nursing homes, adult family homes, halfway houses and homeless missions. There were seven or eight persons with HD. A few patients were seated and others were slowly walking, even pacing to and fro along a side wall. The room was peaceful, with a few quiet conversations between a nurse and a patient, but no talking between patients. There were no particular activities underway. The patients seemed to be simply enveloped in their own little worlds. I knew the families of most of the HD patients because many had previously been seen in our clinic at the university. We reviewed the patients with the staff, and their stories were a revealing survey of how HD can disrupt the lives of ordinary people.

■ ■ ■

Martha was about 45, walking hesitantly and unsteadily with a walker, dressed in black stretch pants and a gray sweatshirt. She had on a red plastic bicycle helmet with a strap under her chin, because of her risk for falls. She smiled and said "Hello," apparently understanding who we were, but did not stop walking. Across the room, Jenny, another middle-aged woman in a brown bathrobe, sat quietly and rigidly at a table, staring at an unfinished jigsaw puzzle. She had occasional twitches of her shoulders and hands. She was making no attempt to work on the puzzle. The staff said she almost never talked but had un-expected temper tantrums.

■ ■ ■

Down the hallway, Gregory, who looked to be in his 20s or 30s, was in his room lying on a mattress pad. In fact, the whole floor was cov-ered with green mattress pads and the walls were lined with similar padding. Gregory wore green hospital pajamas stained with spills from his earlier breakfast. He had severe involuntary movements and could barely stand. The padding was to protect him from injury. He could nod his head, grimace, and speak in monosyllables. The staff had not found a medicine combination that had much effect on his movements. I couldn't help thinking that Gregory was the kind of patient interned at the Hospital Bicetre in Paris at the end of the 18th century and released from chains by Phillipe Pinel and his colleague Jean-Baptiste Pussin. I have no doubt there were patients with HD in that Parisian asylum more than 200 years ago.

■ ■ ■

We also met Sally, whom we had known from our clinic for several years. She was only 23 but had dropped out of high school when she was 16 for "wild behavior." Her mother had died at a young age with HD, and Sally was considered to have juvenile-onset HD with a high CAG repeat number in the gene associated with HD. She had very few involuntary movements but a long list of behavioral problems. She had arrests for drug possession, shoplifting, theft, public drunkenness and exposure. She had chased one of her caretakers with a kitchen knife. This was her third time at Western. On a previous admission she had taken a dislike to another patient and persisted in dumping pitchers of water on his head. Now on medication, she was calm and controlled. She loved cigarettes and was allowed to wander outside on the hospital grounds, chain-smoking and frequently unattended. She even walked to a nearby 7-11 store to buy cigarettes. Surprisingly, she did not run away, although it would have been easy. I think she felt safe at Western and appreciated the compassionate care.

Sally was overweight and sloppily dressed. Although cooperative, she was slow to respond, probably from the sedating effects of medication. In talking with Sally it was apparent that she had trouble telling when the people around her were happy or sad, serious or joking, angry or content. She was unable to "read" another person's facial expressions or emotional modulating of their voice. This difficulty of emotional processing of one's self and others is well recognized in persons with HD. This deficit in emotional recognition has some parallels with autism and with a rare genetic disease called Urbach-Wiethe, in which individuals have degeneration of a specific brain region called the *amygdala*. The amygdala is involved with helping us set our emotional tone and respond to emotions in others, like anger and sadness. This brain area can degenerate in Alzheimer disease and is undoubtedly also affected in HD.

■ ■ ■

Off to the side, sitting alone at a table, I recognized David K, whom we had seen in our clinic several months earlier. Motionless with uncombed, shoulder-length black hair, he stared intensely at the tabletop. He had a curious way of staring that indicated you were not in his world. He was a 25-year-old man with a diagnosis of schizophrenia, but he also had a family history of HD. His psychiatrist had referred him to us to determine if he had HD and, if so, to comment on whether we thought HD was related to his psychosis. In the clinic he sat with both feet up on the chair and his arms wrapped around his knees. We could not generate any conversation from him until we noticed his wristwatch. It was a large, heavy, thick watch, the kind you might find on the wrist of a scuba diver. When we asked him about it he said in a quiet monotone, "It's a special watch. It tells me what to do. It separates good from evil. It tells me to live in a pyramid and then we will all be safe." Apparently this was a parallel world he was living in, where he felt safe under a pyramid listening to his watch. Leaving the topic of his watch and pyramids, we tried to get David to understand genetic testing. He seemed to understand the concept and stated it was fine with him. His test came back positive. In fact, the DNA repeat expansion size was quite large and would fit with an early onset of disease symptoms. Although David had no involuntary movements, I am convinced that his schizophrenic features were a manifestation of a mutation in the gene associated with HD disturbing the equilibrium of his brain. Although frank psychotic features such as delusions and hallucinations are not common in people with HD, they occur more often than expected and are not likely to be a coincidence.

Sitting across the room from David was Connie. She was about the same age as David and had curly, light brown hair. She wore glasses with one cracked lens and was outfitted in an oversized, faded purple University of Washington T-shirt. She was humming quietly and slowly rocking back and forth. Her left hand rested on the table, and with her right hand she held a thick paperback book tightly to her side. The cover was missing and the pages were torn and frayed. She carried the book with her everywhere she went, never letting go. She took it to bed. She had never been seen without it. When asked what she was reading, she responded in a high-pitched, staccato voice: "Oh, nothing special." When we asked if we could take a look at the book, she slowly, tentatively handed it to us. Flipping through the tattered pages we discovered it was *Moby Dick*. We asked, "Do you like this story?" Her high-pitched voice responded, "No, not really." She was much more comfortable when she had the book back in her hand and clutched it snugly to her side. We asked the staff if they had ever seen her reading it. The answer was, "Never." Apparently the book was a comfort object, like a teddy bear, that she constantly hugged and made her feel safe. She certainly needed to feel safe. Her mother had died with HD five or six years before, and Connie had always been lonely and withdrawn, living by herself. Recently, Connie had set fire to her apartment, either in anger or as an attempt to get attention. Today she was quiet, cooperative and passive. One could not have predicted that in four years she would be flagrantly psychotic and delusional with threatening auditory hallucinations.

■ ■ ■

Sitting in an armchair and quietly staring at a television screen was a large man wearing a San Francisco Giants baseball cap. He had a few infrequent twitches of his fingers and occasionally of his whole body. He had been discovered homeless and confused walking near the freeway in Tacoma. Following hospitalization, his story was slowly pieced together. He had been a police officer in Nevada and a

Marine Corps sergeant before that. He mumbled something about Huntington disease in his family and a genetic test proved positive. He had outbursts of anger, could not care for himself, and slowly wound his way through the healthcare system until he reached Western. To control his behavior he was put on fairly high doses of an antipsychotic medication and a tranquilizer. The TV was also a tranquilizer. This approach eliminated his outbursts of anger but resulted in long periods of staring, with almost no social interaction. He did not communicate with the other patients, but he was able to feed himself when the meal tray was brought to him. His coordination was poor, he stumbled when walking, and he broke furniture when he fell. He might eventually be transferred to a nursing home if his behavior remained controlled.

▪ ▪ ▪

Agnes was yet another patient with HD in the mental institution. She had been evicted from three different apartments and had her electricity turned off. She suffered these indignities because she had no money, no social support system and lacked the mental capacity to solve her dilemma. She was left homeless, wandering confused on downtown streets. Picked up by the police, she was eventually shunted to Western. Dr. Lighthouse, the hospital's staff neurologist, said, "She has the worst choreic family history I have ever encountered." Some unknown amateur family genealogist had assembled an extensive record of her ancestors (Figure. 7.2). Agnes' great-great-grandmother had died in an institution in Ohio. Agnes' great-grandfather had died in the South Dakota Lunatic Asylum. Her grandmother had been a patient at Eastern State Hospital near Spokane, Washington. That woman had six children, including Agnes' mother, who had also been a patient at Eastern State. While out on a weekend pass she died in an apartment fire of unknown cause. That woman's brother, Agnes' uncle, had also been a patient with HD at Eastern State Hospital. An aunt died at age 39 with HD in a state hospital in Pennsylvania. Two other uncles had both been patients with HD at Eastern State Hospital and both were moved to the VA Hospital in Tacoma where one died and the other was still alive. The only person in that sibship who did not

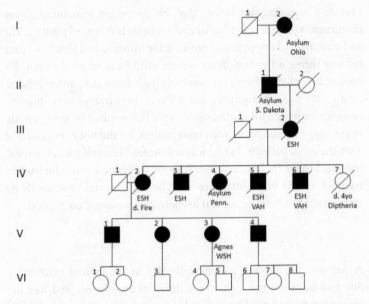

Figure 7.2 ■ "Worst choreic family history." Family pedigree of Agnes (V-3), one of the patients seen at Western State Hospital. Her great-great-grandmother (I-2) died in a mental hospital in Ohio. Her great-grandfather (II-1) died in a mental asylum in South Dakota. Her grandmother (III-2) was in Eastern State Hospital. Agnes' mother (IV-2), aunt and uncles all had Huntington disease (HD) and were in mental institutions. Agnes' sister and two brothers all have HD. There are eight children in the most recent generation (VI) in Agnes' branch of the family, who are each at 50% risk of inheriting HD. There are many more family members not shown on this diagram.

Squares are males, circles are females. Black symbols mean affected with HD. A diagonal line through a symbol indicates deceased. ESH = Eastern State Hospital; WSH = Western State Hospital; VAH = Veterans Affairs Hospital; Penn = Pennsylvania.

have HD was a girl who died at age four with diphtheria. In the next generation, Agnes had two brothers and a sister with HD. Agnes and her siblings all had children who were now at risk for the disease. The family history was indeed impressive and oppressive. The weight of a family history of HD can be a heavy burden pushing down on every generation. In some families, such as this one, the story is clear and intimidating. In other families, the history is glossed over or covered up and the persons with the illness become the proverbial skeletons in the closet.

■ ■ ■

In the two hours I spent on the "Neuro" ward at Western there was no yelling, no screaming; there were no temper tantrums, no seizures, no fights, and no straitjackets. The patients were there because, for one reason or another, no other place would take them. They were getting good care. The hope was that, if it could be documented that they were safe and their behavior controlled on medication, some facility in the community would be able to assume their long-term management. In our conversations with the staff it was clear that the goal of treatment was to discharge the patients following "stabilization" of their behavior. The hospital was overpopulated, understaffed and resources were thin. The days of patients staying at Western for years and decades were mostly over. Sally was an example of the overall failure of the state mental health system. This was her third admission, emblematic of a classic "revolving door" story. On discharge she would eventually stop her medications and not go to her mental health clinic appointments. This would lead to misbehavior, arrest, recognition of her "mental illness" and readmission to Western.

THE ASYLUM MUSEUM AND CEMETERY

When we left the inpatient ward, we discovered that Western has a small hospital museum in the basement with reminders of how some patients with HD used to be treated. Some of the displays are in old, white-tiled rooms closed by heavy, thick doors with peepholes, originally used for the cold-water therapy (a sort of shock therapy often used on mental patients in the 19th and early 20th centuries). Display cases showed an early electroshock machine and a heavy padded straitjacket. The white canvas jacket with long sleeves and a large leather buckle looked deceivingly simple, but obviously effective. It was presumably preferable to metal handcuffs behind the back. (Years ago I had tried on a straitjacket. Comfortable at first, I soon realized I had become an armless man with useless hands and quickly developed a feeling of helpless claustrophobia.) There were also displays describing frontal lobotomy and a "Francis Farmer Room" displaying photos and posters of the Hollywood actress who spent several years at Western in the 1940s.

The friendly, knowledgeable docent described a new national program allowing families to identify relatives who died in asylums and were buried anonymously in the institutional cemeteries. Western has such a plot of land where each grave is marked with a small numbered stone. There are reported to be nearly 3,000 individual plots. If a family believes that a loved one died and was buried at Western, the museum has old records that can match names with grave numbers. This sometimes helps to bring closure to old skeletons in a family closet. I have no doubt that in the first 100 years of Western's history patients with HD ended their lives in the hospital and found their final resting place in a numbered grave.

Soon after returning home from Western State, almost as an unintended reality check, I received the following email message:

Dr. Bird, I need your advice. I am a psychiatrist at our state's only mental hospital. My male patient is 36 years old and was diagnosed with Huntington disease three years ago. His genetic test showed 44 CAG repeats. His father died of the disease after 18 years in an institution. I have had limited experience with this disease. This man is in our forensic unit having a record of more than 10 felony arrests. Although alert and oriented he is often delusional, irritable, angry, and demanding. He frequently refuses medication although I have been trying olanzapine [an antipsychotic drug]. He has required seclusion several times after threatening behavior and physical violence. He has a few jerky movements but plays basketball remarkably well. He "knows" he has HD, but says his behavior outbursts must be caused by something else and demands a CT scan. Can you give me some help in managing this patient?

This note was a stark reminder that mental institutions all over the country continue to struggle with this disease and that there is an important intersection of psychiatry with neurology.

Our field trip to Western State Hospital left us sobered and frustrated by the paradoxes and dilemmas we had just witnessed. Sobered because the patients with HD seemed so compromised and disabled by their disease. Frustrated because the lack of effective treatment was so apparent and the need for a less dreary living environment seemed obvious. Little did we know that the intersection of HD with a psychiatric disaster was about to unfold in an unexpected way.

8

I Don't Know Why I Did It

The phone call came from an individual who identified himself as a public defender for King County Superior Court. He related that he had been assigned the case of George, a 20-year-old man who was charged with murder. He was calling me because the man came from a family with Huntington disease and it was realized that he was at risk for this brain disease. The attorney stated that he had been reading about HD and discovered that this was a disease in which the top and the middle of the brain deteriorated and left the bottom of the brain intact. Furthermore, he had read that the bottom of the brain was called the "reptilian brain" and he thought perhaps this could be the basis of a defense, sort of "his reptile brain made him do it." He wanted to know what I thought of this idea and if I could determine whether or not the young man had HD. The thought of a "horned toad defense" passed through my mind and I told him I thought the reptilian brain defense was not a good idea. I said we certainly could see the man in our clinic and give a diagnostic determination.

The following week, two quiet, burly King County Jail policemen brought George to our clinic, hand-cuffed and in an orange jumpsuit. The records from the public defender's office outlined his story. He had graduated from high school with weak but passing grades in special education. His IQ had been measured as 100 ("normal") and he was said to be dyslexic. He was a loner, didn't socialize, and had accumulated a police record for petty larceny, criminal trespass, and marijuana possession. His mother had died at age 32 with a diagnosis of HD. He had had a few odd jobs but was mostly unemployed. He was living in a small, dilapidated rental house with another unemployed man he had met in a park. One day, while they were watching television, George pulled a .38 caliber handgun from his jacket pocket, turned in his chair, and shot and killed his roommate. He wandered outside and threw the gun into the underbrush. He then left the scene and went to his father's house, saying nothing about the incident.

Meanwhile, the shots had been heard and the police were called. They found the dead roommate, quickly located the discarded gun, and identified the name of the missing roommate. They drove to George's father's house, where they found him watching TV. They read him his rights and he quickly confessed to the crime. When asked his motivation he said, "I don't know why I did it. I just felt the urge." On more detailed questioning over the next several days he never gave a different explanation. His lack of empathy was profound.

The most remarkable thing about his examination in the clinic was that he had absolutely none of the involuntary jerky movements one might expect in a person with HD. He sat quietly and had nothing much to say. In fact, he was withdrawn, had no emotional tone and appeared very apathetic. George unnervingly just stared ahead and seemed disinterested. He had a "thousand mile stare"—distant, distracted and disconnected.[1] George spoke only when spoken to and then in only one- or two-word responses. His thinking seemed very concrete, unable to make connections or express ideas. He denied having hallucinations or delusions. He gave no information about his roommate, his family, his part-time jobs, or his experiences in school.

These were the days before the availability of a genetic blood test for HD, but we decided to do two other tests paid for by the county. The first was a brain MRI. This sometimes can reveal atrophy of the caudate nucleus deep in the brain, the area first affected by HD (see Figures 1.2 and 1.3). However, the brain MRI is often normal early in the course of the disease. His MRI was normal. We also obtained an electroencephalogram (EEG) brain-wave test to see if there was any evidence of a seizure or other subtle brain abnormalities. This, too, was normal.

We eventually obtained the medical record for his mother, who indeed had the diagnosis of HD. She had died in her 30s with typical characteristics of the disease, including abnormal movements.

I told the public defender that my best educated guess was that George probably did have HD, as poor judgment, lack of impulse control, confusion, and massive apathy can be part of the disease. Furthermore, the age of onset of symptoms has a tendency to be roughly similar within families and it was significant that his mother had developed HD and died of the disease at a relatively young age. On the other hand, his lack of abnormal movements, normal MRI, and the unavailability of a specific diagnostic test left the final diagnosis somewhat in question.

George was later found guilty of second-degree homicide with no evidence of premeditation and sent to the state prison in the nearby town of Monroe.

Six years later, I received a phone call from the Monroe Prison psychologist. He said he had recently evaluated George and reviewed his record. He wanted to let me know that this 26-year-old man now had definite involuntary movements. He wondered if our clinic could see him again because, in the intervening years, the genetic blood test for the mutation causing HD had become available. Of course we could.

The second time around, George had changed. This time, although still dressed in an orange jumpsuit, he was in a wheelchair and not handcuffed. He was the same withdrawn man of few words that we remembered from before, but he now had definite sudden jumps and jerks of his shoulders and hands, although not severe or disabling. Furthermore, he was quite stiff and rigid and could barely walk. Although he looked a bit like a young man with Parkinson disease, these dramatic changes made it clear that he did indeed have HD. We also confirmed this with a genetic blood test. He had 53 CAG repeats in the gene associated with HD. Not only was this result abnormal, but his DNA expansion was even higher than that found in the typical person with HD. This fit with the relatively early onset of his symptoms and those of his mother, from whom he must have inherited the mutation.

With this diagnosis confirmed and his disability progressing, George was released from prison and sent to a group home. He was felt to be of no risk for violence or escape, and the Monroe Prison, like the Walla Walla Penitentiary, was full. We saw him one more time and he appeared to be well cared for. He died about three years later.

HOW WAS GEORGE'S BRAIN DISCONNECTED?

The story of George is sad and perplexing. Most persons with HD do not commit violent crimes. And yet I believe his brain disease was very much involved with his behavior. Unfortunately, he had never given a clue that he might suddenly act out with this strange behavior. He had never seen a psychiatrist and was on no medication. It probably was not difficult for him to purchase a handgun. We will never know why he thought he needed one, and can only wish it was not so readily available.

It seems certain that George's impulsive and destructive behavior was directly related to the deterioration of his brain caused by HD and likely concentrated in his frontal lobes.

The abnormal behavior associated with damage to the frontal lobes of the brain is well recognized. One of the earliest descriptions is said to have been that of Phineas Gage. Phineas was the infamous mid-19th-century Vermont railroad worker who was tamping dynamite into rocks with a metal rod when a sudden explosion blew the rod through the front of his skull. Surprisingly, he eventually recovered and was able to walk, talk, and even return to a different job. He was initially reported to have had a dramatic change in his personality and behavior, becoming unpredictable, obstreperous and no longer the same old Phineas. There is little actual documentation of his personality change, and apparently there was considerable slow improvement. Nevertheless, 100 years later, with the use of frontal lobotomies to treat psychiatric disease, it has become clear that personalities can be dramatically changed by the operation. A frontal lobotomy is the surgical equivalent of what happened accidentally to Phineas Gage, except the operation includes both frontal lobes. Apathy and lack of initiative are especially common. Impulsivity also occurs, but not specifically related to violent behavior. In thinking about these examples of damage to the frontal lobes, I have been struck how patients with HD are often similar to those with another degenerative brain disease, frontotemporal dementia (FTD) (see Chapter 2). Lack of impulse control, antisocial behavior, apathy, and unexpected and strange behaviors all occur in both diseases. It is not difficult to imagine these same kinds of mechanisms being involved in a wide variety of mental illnesses. George's frontal lobes were badly disrupted by HD and the results were disastrous.

Perhaps what happened to George is what happened in the case of Dr. Vince Gilmer. Dr. Gilmer's story was highlighted in an episode of "This American Life" on National Public Radio in 2013.[2,3] Dr. Gilmer was a successful and popular general practitioner in a small North Carolina town in the 1990s. Suddenly, and without any apparent explanation, he strangled and killed his father. Dr. Gilmer defended himself at his own trial with a rambling defense about a chemical serotonin imbalance in his brain. Jurors thought he was some kind of malingerer, found him guilty of murder, and sentenced him to life in prison. Ten years later his strange story was investigated by the physician who took over his practice, oddly and coincidentally also named Dr. Gilmer (Ben instead of Vince). He discovered that his predecessor's father had been hospitalized many years before with a diagnosis of schizophrenia. Released from the mental hospital, the father and son had gotten into a violent argument and the son suddenly strangled his father, leading to the son's trial and prison sentence. While in prison, Dr. Gilmer, the criminal, had developed chorea. He was eventually discovered to have HD, documented by a genetic blood test showing the mutation. It seems very likely his father also had HD rather than schizophrenia—a remarkable turn of events.

Commentators have quickly noted that it should not be assumed that HD "caused" Dr. Gilmer to murder his father. This is certainly true, because such sudden violent acts are not common in persons with HD. The occasional violence I have seen perpetrated by persons with HD is rarely premeditated and usually associated with sudden impulsivity, the so-called disinhibition associated with brain damage. Nevertheless, I would argue that HD is playing a role in such cases and is an important contributing factor. This is not only an important biological issue but also has societal implications. The extensive arguments for and against using evidence of brain damage or brain disease in criminal trials is beyond the scope of this book and has been reviewed in excellent detail by Kevin Davis in *The Brain Defense*.[4] If not used in the guilt phase of a trial, it seems reasonable that evidence of a serious brain disease is appropriate in the punishment phase. In my opinion, people like George and Vince Gilmer should be maintained and cared for in a locked psychiatric facility, for life if necessary, rather than warehoused in a prison with no medical or psychiatric treatment.

The disinhibition and profound lack of empathy demonstrated by George is reminiscent of another young man seen in our clinic. His behavior was essentially uncontrollable. He was constantly threatening his father, older sister, and her young child with physical harm and had actually attacked a family member and threatened another with a knife. He abused alcohol and methadone and was frequently arrested by the police. He usually bounced from jail to a juvenile detention center to a brief inpatient stay in a psychiatric facility. He had run away from numerous detention centers, only to be recaptured when he got into a fight or overdosed on drugs and alcohol. Because he had no movement disorder there was considerable discussion at to whether his behavior was actually a manifestation of HD or just that of a misbehaving adolescent. Although his result was outside the "normal" range, the CAG repeat expansion size did not fall into the unusually large range seen with juvenile HD. On the other hand, his father noted that his aggressive behavior and physical violence were "identical" to that of his mother, who had died at age 45 with symptomatic HD (their genetic test results were identical). It was remarkable that in interviews he was perfectly calm, emotionally detached, and expressed no remorse for his behavior or concern for those he had threatened or attacked. He seemed to fit into a category variously referred to in the adolescent psychiatry literature as "conduct disorder" or "oppositional defiant disorder" or "antisocial personality disorder associated with callous/unemotional traits."[5] Young persons with these conditions are often aggressive, show rule violation behavior, and are impulsive and unemotional. Another man with HD and similar behavior so frightened his 78-year-old grandmother that she bought a Taser gun for protection. Individuals with this syndrome may have a defect in the amygdala, a brain region associated with empathy and fear, although the biological basis of the behavior is surely complicated. Little is known about the neurological deficits in such persons, and it is of considerable interest that the constellation of findings can be found in some individuals with HD.

Violence in the world of HD can also work in the opposite direction. That is, the person with HD becomes the victim in the violent edges of society, as we shall see in the next chapter.

References

1. Reiswig G. *Thousand Mile Stare: One Family's Journey through the Struggle and Science of Alzheimer's*. Nicholas Brealey, London, 2010.
2. Blake C. Saving Dr. Gilmer, *Asheville NC Citizen Times*, May 25, 2013.
3. Koenig S. "Dr. Gilmer and Mr. Hyde." *This American Life*. April 12, 2013. https://www.thisamericanlife.org/492/dr-gilmer-and-mr-hyde.
4. Davis K. *The Brain Defense: Murder in Manhattan and the Dawn of Neuroscience in the Courtroom*. Penguin Press, New York, 2014.
5. Blair RJR, Leibenluft E, Pine DS. Conduct disorder and callous-unemotional traits in youth. *New England Journal of Medicine*, 371:2207–16, 2014.

9

Carkeek Park

Carkeek Park is a lovely, green Pacific Coast park nestled in the northwest corner of Seattle (Figure 9.1). It is a small second-growth forest of tall Douglas fir and cedar mixed with alder and maple that gently slopes down to a quiet waterfront area on Puget Sound. There is an old apple orchard on the property and several miles of trails winding through the quiet woods. On a wet summer day in 2003, a solemn work detail from the Seattle Police Department arrived in a heavy northwest mist and began digging in the turf 50 yards or so off one of the trails. A man in handcuffs had led them to the spot. The ground was rain soaked, so digging was easy. They were looking for a grave. Two feet down, they found the body of Bobby Thomas, one of our former patients with HD.

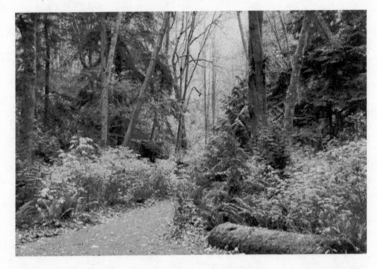

Figure 9.1 ■ Carkeek Park, in the northwest corner of Seattle. The body of a man with Huntington disease was discovered buried here.

The case was described like this by Ian Ith, in the *Seattle Times* (quoted with permission)[1]:

Roommate Held in Death of Man with Huntington's

Bobby Thomas had Huntington's disease, a crippling fatal nervous-system disorder that he did everything he could to cope with – and often pretended to ignore, his mother said.

The 33 year old Thomas did drugs, drank, and rebelled to numb the depression of knowing he would die young, said his mother. But Thomas was a trusting soul who looked to anyone for approval, even if they were the wrong kinds of people, she said.

Now police say they believe one of those people – Brian Roberts, Thomas' 23 year old roommate – broke the disabled man's neck and strangled him several months ago. He allegedly let Thomas' body languish in a closet for days, then wheeled it in a recycling bin to Seattle's Carkeek Park, where he buried it in a makeshift grave in the woods, according to documents filed this week in King County Superior Court.

Now Thomas' mother says she is relieved that a suspect is in jail, awaiting formal charges later this week. But she said she still wonders how someone could have taken advantage of someone so physically helpless.

"It's so horrible for him to have suffered," she said. "Not only was he killed, but part of his whole entire family was killed, and will never be the same."

Yesterday, Roberts remained held in the King County Jail on $500,000 bail, on a separate charge of attacking a new roommate with a machete earlier this month. Police say that attack ended up linking Roberts to Thomas' slaying, which likely happened sometime before April.

Though Roberts has not formally been charged, police spelled out some of the case against him in an application for a search warrant filed in King County Superior Court. The documents say police took carpet samples and found hair and a button in the closet of the Greenwood apartment where Thomas' body had been stored.

Police unearthed Thomas' remains off a trail in the wooded park July 4th after Roberts led them to the spot, court documents say.

Police had been looking for Thomas since early May, when his mother called to say she had not heard from her son for several weeks and he had not been collecting his medical-benefits checks.

Thomas was born and raised in Seattle and attended high school before dropping out about the same time his father died of Huntington's disease, a hereditary, degenerative brain disorder that eventually robs a person of the most basic functions of movement and thinking.

Thomas soon would begin to exhibit signs of the disease, as would his sister, who is now in a nursing home. "He couldn't understand her. He started crying," his friend said of the two siblings who shared the fatal genetic disease. The degenerative disorder had affected his sister's speech. "Bobby had seen his dad die from it. He was pretty depressed. He knew he was next."

Thomas spent time in trouble with the law, in and out of jails, hospitals, camps, group homes, his mother said. About a year ago, he decided to move back to Seattle from California to live with friends. He thought he might be able pick up odd jobs, but the *living arrangements were not what were promised and the job never materialized.*

It wasn't clear how he met Roberts, but eventually Thomas, by then a tall gaunt man who had trouble moving and walking, moved in with Roberts at an apartment less than 10 blocks from Carkeek Park.

His mother said she last heard from her son when he called in mid-March. Seattle police detectives had found some of Thomas' friends, one of whom said he figured Thomas was dead, police documents say.

On July 3, Roberts was arrested on suspicion of using a machete to hack the arm of a new roommate, a 31 year old man who had moved into Thomas' old room. Court documents say the two men got in an argument while watching a video and Roberts grabbed the long blade off a coffee table.

While talking to police, the new roommate revealed that Roberts had broken Thomas' neck during a fight, then strangled him with a phone cord. Roberts claimed Thomas "came into his bedroom and attacked him." Roberts stashed the body in the closet, but when it began to decompose and smell, he used a recycling bin to transport it to Carkeek Park.

After taking the body to Carkeek Park, he then hid the recycling bin in the apartment closet. But when the new roommate moved into Thomas' room in late April, Roberts ripped up the carpet from the closet, put it in the bin, and wheeled it all to the park to leave it not far from Thomas' grave.

Police say they questioned Roberts, who then agreed to take them to the park and show them where to dig. Roberts' criminal record consists of three assault charges in 1995, when he was about 15. They were eventually dismissed after he completed diversion programs through juvenile court in King County.

Brian Roberts was found guilty of second-degree homicide and sentenced to 38 years in prison. It was second degree because no premeditation could be proven and he claimed Bobby had attacked him first.

This story obviously stands in stark contrast to that of George in Chapter 8. George was a man with HD who killed his roommate. Bobby was a man with HD who was killed by his roommate. Bobby's case has more facts to work with than George's story, but it still requires some speculation. He certainly used poor judgment in selecting a roommate; impaired judgment is a common characteristic of HD. He probably was impulsive and we know that he had a history of drug use and petty crimes. Impulsivity is common in HD as well. Bobby was also depressed about his father, his sister and his own diagnosis. It is possible he picked a fight with his roommate, but there is no way to be certain. Finally, we do know that he had chorea and poor coordination, which left him physically vulnerable to an attacker. When persons with HD have this collection of symptoms (poor judgment, impulsivity, depression, chorea and incoordination) they become classic "disasters waiting to happen." Without a strong support group and a safe caring environment, they can get into big trouble very fast. We will see an example of this trouble in the next chapter.

Reference

1. Ith I. Roommate held in the death of man with Huntington's. *Seattle Times*, July 16 2003.

10

Please Call the Coroner

The woman's voice on the telephone sounded hurried, but forceful and clear. "My name is Megan Brown. You probably don't remember us, but you saw our family years ago. My sister had Huntington's disease. I tested normal, but she died a few years later. I am asking you to please call the county coroner. My nephew, my sister's son, was shot and killed by the police two weeks ago. You never saw him, but we in the family thought it was real important that his blood get tested for the Huntington's because he has a three-year-old daughter. We told the coroner to save his blood for the test and he said he would. Will you please do this for us? It's real important to the family. When she is older that little girl will need to know if she is at risk for the Huntington's or not. Please call the coroner right away."

Needless to say, this was uncharted territory for us. I tried to get more information from Megan but there wasn't much. Her nephew was 25 and had a history of drug problems. He had been in jail and released a few weeks before. She said he was running away from the police and they shot him. She did not know why he was running, nor why the police felt obligated to shoot him. I don't know how much more she knew, but I was unable to discover any further details. I told her the least I could do was check the story with the coroner and get back to her.

Checking the clinic file confirmed the family information. I had seen them several years ago and Megan's sister had fairly advanced HD. Megan had a normal genetic test for HD and her sister with the disease had a small son. This boy was now obviously the young man who had just been shot and killed.

The county coroner was straightforward, matter-of-fact, and co-operative. He confirmed the man had been shot and was now his coroner's case. He also confirmed that the family requested he save blood samples for a genetic test and he had done so. He knew nothing about the name of the test or what lab would perform it, but if I wanted to take on that task he would send the sample to any certified lab that I directed him to.

The appropriate legal or ethical aspects of this case were not clear to me, but I called the University Hospital genetics lab and explained the situation. After an internal discussion they told me if they received the sample and I was the ordering doctor, they would run the test. The lab director wanted to know who would pay for the test and who would get the result. I said the result would be sent to me, I would determine who was going to pay for it, and I also needed to determine who in the family would be informed of the result.

I called Megan back and described my conversations with the coroner and the lab. She said she would pay the $250 for the test. Her nephew really did not have a close next-of-kin. His mother had died of HD. His father had disappeared and no one knew his whereabouts. The nephew was divorced and had no contact with his ex-wife. His only child was the three-year-old daughter. Megan said either she would make the long drive into Seattle to obtain the test result or she would find a blood relative living closer willing to take on that task.

As luck would have it, three weeks later the deceased nephew's sister arrived in the clinic for a follow-up visit that had been scheduled almost a year before. It became clear that she was fully aware of the situation in the family and knew that her brother had been shot and killed by the police. She said that she knew nothing more about the circumstances, but said she specifically wished to have her brother's test result given to her. She had already discussed this with other members of the family and she had become the family "point person."

The test result returned and indeed the young dead man had the mutation for HD. Somehow this was not a complete surprise. His drug and jail problems may well have been a clue. In any event, his daughter was now at 50% risk, just as he had been.

The sister was saddened and tearful with her brother's news. She herself was an asymptomatic person who knew she had inherited the mutation for HD. Her brother's result was yet another burden for her and her family.

Many months later we discovered more information about the man who had been shot. He had been a loner and social misfit as an adolescent, followed by a long history of assault, burglary, drug abuse and attempted rape. His motto was visibly tattooed high on his neck: "Fuck the World."[1] On one occasion, following a burglary, he climbed a tree and taunted the police to come after him, which they did. More recently he was on probation from serving several years in prison for second-degree assault. He had broken probation and, when he saw US marshals coming to arrest him, he pulled a gun and fired a shot. The marshals returned fire and killed him. One can only wonder what role HD played in his life of anger and antisocial behavior. He had been raised by a mother with symptomatic HD (whose mother, in turn, we discovered had been at Western State Hospital), and the abnormal HD protein had been working its destruction on his brain for years. His story has many parallels with that of George in Chapter 8 who killed his roommate.

To this day, I do not know if we followed the correct strategy in trying to help this family. It seemed perfectly reasonable for the family to wonder if the man had HD because they were worried about his daughter's risk. In fact, it seemed like quick thinking to request the coroner to save the blood. Should the blood have been banked and not tested? Who would have "owned" the sample? Should the blood have been discarded and never tested? Who was the legal next-of-kin? When will his daughter be told she is at risk? Who will tell her? Should an attorney have been hired to sort this all out? Could it have been sorted out? Would the end result have ultimately been the same as it had actually played out?

The years have passed and we have heard nothing more from the family. Eventually, we probably will.

In many ways this scenario was similar to the strategy we used before the discovery of the HD gene. With the consent of patients and their families, we saved blood samples from persons with the clinical diagnosis of HD. This was done on the assumption that, even after the patient's death, we would be able to confirm the diagnosis at the genetic level following the discovery of the gene and the availability of a diagnostic DNA test. This actually has come to pass in a number of situations and was very helpful to future generations of several families. In every instance I can remember the genetic test confirmed the older clinical diagnosis.

We will now turn to some coping strategies that are much more successful than battling with the police.

Reference

1. Hoke C. *Wanted: A Spiritual Pursuit Through Jail, Among Outlaws, and Across Borders*. HarperOne, New York, 2015, p. 367.

PART II

Coping Strategies

Individuals with symptomatic Huntington disease and their families develop a variety of mechanisms for coping with their difficult circumstances. Dance, music, travel, sports, service animals and social engagement can all be employed in successful ways.

Onset of HD in childhood, although uncommon, is one of the greatest challenges for a family. This is called "juvenile HD" and when it occurs, family members, teachers, and childhood friends can form an important supportive social network for the affected child. We will meet a "princess in pink" who was fortunate enough to be surrounded by such a network.

Because there is no cure for HD, or even a treatment that slows disease progression, it is not surprising that families with HD often try a variety of unproven remedies. In this section we will hear the story of a man who had an unusual experience with magnetic brain stimulation.

Suicide is an "end-game" strategy that is commonly discussed and greatly feared in the HD community. Tremendous effort can be applied to its prevention, but even the best efforts are sometimes defeated.

It is also important to recognize that persons who have inherited the mutation for HD can have happy, productive and successful lives for many years before they develop advanced symptoms. This is especially true for individuals who have onset of symptoms late in life.

Of course, having HD does not protect the affected person from developing other diseases. A second diagnosis of another equally devastating disease can seriously challenge one's coping mechanisms.

The following stories will touch on all these complex aspects of coping with HD.

11

Enjoy the Moment

Mary was 45 years old when she decided to have genetic testing. Her mother had died with HD and her brother was living in another state with fairly advanced symptoms. She herself had no symptoms, a normal physical exam, and was employed by the University of Washington. She liked her niche job, which involved helping college students find housing. Her genetic test results demonstrated the mutation associated with HD; she had inherited the mutation from her mother. She took the results with a sigh but seemed neither upset nor depressed. Her attitude was that the test was simply one of those unfortunate breaks, that she felt "normal" and that she needed to get on with her busy life. Keeping busy was a good way to cope. She had a companion who was very helpful and supportive.

The next year, I asked Mary if she would discuss her experience with genetic testing as part of my annual lecture on genetic testing to second-year medical student class. It was always instructive to have a real-live person discuss the experience of pursuing genetic testing for HD and answer the student's questions. The lecture could be intimidating for the patient because he or she sat with me in front of a class 150 inquisitive students staring down from 15 tiered rows of desks in a large lecture hall.

Mary was a star in this centuries-old tradition of medical theater-in-the round. Unfazed, she calmly described her family, why she decided to proceed with testing, and how she felt about the positive results. A student asked her if she found any benefit from the testing. Mary paused, and then said, "Yes. I always thought that when I retired I would take up dancing. The positive genetic test made me decide not to wait. I have been taking dancing lessons and I love it. It is good for my body and good for my soul. I am glad that I didn't postpone my dancing and I see this as a real unexpected benefit of the testing." The students broke into spontaneous applause. A few months later I attended an HD fund-raising event that featured a lively western band. I caught sight of Mary gracefully gliding around the dance floor, a look of joy and contentment on her face. For the moment she seemed to have found a comfortable equilibrium in her life, somehow balancing her love of dancing with her HD dilemma.

■ ■ ■

Jenny was 42 and had symptomatic HD. She lived in an apartment by herself. I thought she might be lonely, but she had many friends, kept busy and had an upbeat, bubbly, positive attitude, almost manic. She was tall, solidly built and probably had been a good athlete in her younger days. Now it was hard for her to sit still because of her jumpy movements. Her speech was slurred and her walking was unsteady. One day her clinic visit began with my usual question, "How are you doing?" She laughed and nearly shouted, "I am Texas line-dancing! Want to see me do it?" There was no need for a response because she immediately jumped up, began to hum a tune and dance right there in the clinic exam room, her ponytail bouncing up and down like a teenager's. She wasn't falling and was surprisingly nimble on her feet. "Come on and join me," she said. So there we were, a nurse, two neurologists, a genetics counselor, and Jenny doing a little Texas two-step. She was the best dancer of the group and we all laughed. With a mischievous gleam she said, "Look, I'm on YouTube!" She pulled out her iPhone, pressed a few buttons, and showed us a video of a group of people Texas line-dancing in a tavern. There was Jenny in the middle of the group, clapping and swaying with everyone else. The joy was obvious and HD had been forgotten, at least for awhile.

■ ■ ■

Mimi was 75 and also had HD. She had late onset of symptoms. In her early 70s her family physician had noted unexpected, constant, jerky movements. He remembered HD from his medical-school days and obtained the genetic test. Surprising to everyone, the test came back showing the HD mutation. The CAG expansion number was relatively low, but still in the abnormal range. This is commonly the result found in persons who have a delayed, late onset of symptoms. Mimi's husband and children were greatly distressed. Mimi, on the other hand, was unflappable and seemed unconcerned about the result. She had other things to do and tried to lead her usual, busy, energetic life. In fact, she began to focus on her Jazzercise class as the highlight of her day. She had three classes a week, always looked forward to them, and could not stop talking about them. She, too, was happy to demonstrate her Jazzercise steps in the exam room. She would get very excited and her eyes would glow whenever Jazzercise was mentioned. Mimi was short, thin and a bundle of energy. I could picture her in powder-blue tights and pink sneakers as she bounced to the music in her class, but we were afraid that she was so energetic that she might fall and break a hip. A call to her class instructor confirmed that she was aware of Mimi's disease and carefully monitored her activities. Her classmates enjoyed her enthusiasm and were motivated by her upbeat enthusiasm.

■ ■ ■

Susan was 58 and also had the genetic mutation for HD. She had no physical symptoms—no jumps, no jerks, no involuntary movements of any kind. For many years she had been seeing a psychiatrist for a diagnosis of bipolar disorder and she also had an attraction to alcohol. Her outlet in life was bowling. She belonged to a league, bowled twice a week, and enjoyed telling us her average and latest best score. It seemed to be a great outlet for both her physical and emotional needs.

■ ■ ■

These four women nicely illustrate the success of a pleasant-activities strategy in the lives of persons struggling with a progressing brain disease and a serious, often depressing diagnosis. Find something you like to do and do it. Enjoy it. Add a pinch of pleasure to your life.

This formula also worked for Gordon Redfield, at least for a while. Mr. Redfield was a retired banker. He retired not because of HD but because he had a successful 30-year career and wanted to enjoy his senior years. He and his wife traveled, but he got special enjoyment from playing softball. He played for a senior men's team and was one of the best outfielders. When we saw him in the clinic for the first time he clearly had symptomatic HD. Nothing severe, but he had involuntary movements, a jerky speech pattern and could not walk a straight line. Somehow none of this interfered with his softball. Neat and tidy with carefully combed hair, not surprising for a retired banker, he usually wore shorts, a T-shirt and running shoes, ready for action. Short, thin and muscular he excitedly described his catches in the field and his hits at bat. He was getting maximum pleasure out of an activity that he thoroughly enjoyed. Eventually, his HD caught up with him. He became so disabled that he had to stop both softball and driving. He shook his head in despair that he had to give up both. Going from bad to worse, his wife died of cancer shortly thereafter and he was forced to leave his home and move into an assisted living facility. He became a very unhappy man, and our clinic team all tried our very best to ease his depression. We always remember Mr. Redfield as our cheery, softball playing banker.

■ ■ ■

Stanley has had symptoms of HD for more than a dozen years. He lost his job as a carpenter and is now dependent on his wife for even simple tasks of daily living. He cannot walk without falling so spends most his time in a wheelchair. His "savior" is Charlie, his golden retriever. Stanley and Charlie go everywhere together and have perfectly bonded. We have watched them maneuver the halls together as a happy team, Stanley's hand on Charlie's back. They are buddies. Stanley's ability to cope with HD is immensely improved by having Charlie around.

■ ■ ■

Tim Bennett's coping skills were severely tested when his life trajectory hit a sudden, dramatic and surprising curve. He was a school teacher and fourth grade was his specialty. His daily engagement with 25 exuberant children was the great and rewarding challenge of his life. He was especially pleased that he had the same kids for two years because he would teach fourth grade, then fifth grade, then start over again. Most people would be exhausted by a roomful of 9- and 10-year-olds, but Tim was a master at controlling and focusing their attention.

The shadow of HD loomed in Tim's past, but he was initially unbothered by it. His father had been a successful traveling salesman. However, in his 50s, his business began to unravel. He became confused and had trouble keeping track of finances. His coordination deteriorated. He became more and more clumsy. His doctors were puzzled for several years until the family heard that his sister, Tim's aunt, living in another city, had been given the diagnosis of HD. Tim's father was tested and, sure enough, he too had HD. His physical and mental condition slowly and relentlessly deteriorated. He died in an assisted living facility in his early 70s.

In his late 40s Tim became concerned that his mind was not functioning quite right. He had trouble accurately describing this feeling, but he said his head felt "cloudy." He worried that this could be an early sign of HD and sought counseling. His evaluation was entirely normal, but he decided to proceed with genetic testing. The result was positive. He had inherited the HD mutation from his father. He was not surprised, having already decided that this would be the result.

He also was not depressed by his HD test. Instead, he became proactive. He joined the local HD support group and campaigned to increase community awareness of this disease. He also had no trouble continuing his teaching. His favorite adventure was taking his students on field trips to a lovely nearby local lake surrounded by towering cedar and hemlock. They collected a wild assortment of bugs and plants, brought them back to the classroom, and put them in a glass-enclosed aquarium box. They carefully watched and inspected their collection over the next several weeks. Tim loved stimulating their curiosity. One year he took his class on an overnight trip to visit the massive Grand Coulee Dam, on the Columbia River in Eastern Washington. He recalls seeing a video in the visitor's center of Woody Guthrie singing his famous folk songs from the 1930s. With a twinge of anxiety, he remembered that Woody had died with HD.

Time rolled along without complications until about eight years after receiving his genetic test result. Tim began to notice little muscle twitches in his left arm. His arm never moved. Instead, these were barely noticeable, tiny contractions of a single muscle lasting less than a second. A few weeks later he noticed similar twitches in his shoulder. These little muscle blips were annoying, but not troubling. A few months later, however, he noticed his left hand was getting clumsy. In fact, one day he had to ask his son to help him tie his necktie. He asked his family doctor about these symptoms and was referred to a neurologist. The neurologist said he needed an electromyogram (EMG). An EMG uses tiny needles to electronically measure muscle activity throughout the body. Tim's EMG revealed abnormal twitches in almost every muscle. The neurologist said that Tim's physical examination, symptoms, and EMG results unfortunately all led to the diagnosis of ALS, or Lou Gehrig's disease.

Tim was shocked. He had heard of ALS and the famous ice-bucket challenge fund-raising event that had swamped the Internet. He knew it was an incurable and fatal disease. He asked for a second opinion and got the same answer: he had ALS.

It took a few weeks for Tim to adjust to this devastating news. In the back of his mind he had been expecting to eventually deal with HD and now, suddenly, he had to contend with a completely new and even more rapidly progressive neurological disease. After careful reflection, his attitude did not change. He joined the local ALS support group and became a vigorous community spokesman for his new disease. Meanwhile, his ALS proved to be quite aggressive. His right hand soon became weak and then both legs. After six months he stopped teaching and became confined to a chair in his home. His school organized a wonderful public celebration of his 27-year teaching career. There were lots of balloons and moving tributes to his excellence as a teacher. Many of his past students dropped by to tell him how much they appreciated his impact on their lives.

The ALS began to affect Tim's speech and swallowing. He used a microphone for speech enhancement and was learning to spell words using eye movements on a special electronic screen. His paralysis made it impossible to know if he was developing the choreic movements of HD, although he was about the same age as when his father developed symptoms. Tim's son and sister became his 24/7 caregivers, allowing him to remain at home. His sister carefully searched the Internet, looking for someone else who had both HD and ALS. No one was found. Tim was apparently the only person in the world with both diseases, not a world record anyone would want.

When asked how he felt about this double diagnosis, Tim said he had no regrets. He had enjoyed a full and productive life and was especially proud of his teaching. In fact, he felt that his positive HD genetic test had helped him deal with his later diagnosis of ALS. For years he had mentally prepared to eventually deal with a progressive, degenerative neurological disease. That the disease turned out to be ALS rather than HD was a surprise, but he was able to make the shift. His resilience in the face of these two misfortunes was truly admirable.

■ ■ ■

One of the important points of this chapter is that HD is not just about psychosis and violence and depression and suicide. It is easy to focus on dramatic and unsettling cases displaying these often disturbing elements. But many persons with HD have rewarding and interesting lives filled with the simple pleasures that can be so important. If the disease is going to last 15 or 20 years, there is time to enjoy the moment, at least in the early stages. Carolyn, in the next chapter, was also able to do just this.

12

High Five

I am at the clinic and here comes Carolyn. Her cup is half-full and she always has a smile on her freckled face. She has unquenchable good humor and leaves a trail of smiles as she sways through the clinic lobby. She bustles into the room with a laugh and always seems slightly out of breath as if she just had an exciting experience that she needs to quickly relate. Her mother, grandfather, uncle and two cousins have all died with HD. She lost her job because of problems with her coordination and has since been unemployed. None of that has kept her from being upbeat. She likes to tell the story that her first symptom was involuntary tapping of her foot. With her lovely voice she sang in a barbershop quartet. The repetitive tapping of her foot bothered the director and he told her to stop it. The tapping was not in rhythm and it was annoying the other singers. At the time, she had no idea of the ominous nature of these movements. Now she sees the irony and, recalling her director's impatience, she bursts out laughing when she tells the story.

She dances jerkily into the clinic exam room and wants to show me the new "HD high five." When I go to slap her raised right hand she misses on purpose and hits me on the shoulder. To much laughter she wants to do it twice more with the same uncoordinated, sloppy result. The following year, when she and her sister described her family story and her disease to 150 rapt medical students, she ended by doing the HD high five with me. The students laughed and were obviously touched.

Carolyn and her sister also like to tell the story of when they were traveling in Vancouver, Canada, and she clumsily dropped an expensive bottle of Scotch that they had purchased as a gift for the sister's husband. Smelling of booze, staggering with her HD gait and with slurred speech, they hailed a taxi and tried to explain that Carolyn wasn't drunk. The cabbie didn't buy her excuse, but nonchalantly sprayed the back seat with room deodorant, waved them in and off they went. Her sister says, "You laugh or you cry. It is your choice. We prefer laughter."

Carolyn lived with her sister and not only were they dealing with her HD, but they were caring for their father with Alzheimer disease. Their positive attitude and coping skills were phenomenal.

Carolyn's HD slowly but relentlessly progressed. Last time I saw her she could no longer walk and was in a nursing home. She could still smile. Her sister said she could look back on the good times and keep moving forward. Carolyn's supportive family kept her safe and, along with Social Security Disability funds, kept her financially solvent. Unlike many persons with HD, Carolyn was never depressed. On the other hand, depression became a big problem for Albert, whom we will meet in the next chapter.

13

Let's Try a Magnet

"Albert, you need to take some time off, get some rest and see your doctor." This was not the message Albert wanted to hear, but he was worried and knew his law partner was trying to be helpful and had his best interests at heart.

Albert Sullivan was a highly successful attorney. His wife described him as having a type A personality. She meant this as a compliment. It was why he was so successful. That characteristic also flowed over into his personal life. He was a marathoner and a mountain climber. He liked challenges. When he turned 65 he had no interest in contemplating retirement.

However, when Albert reached 70 his high-strung personality began to change into a heightened sense of anxiety that he could no longer control. He began to worry about everything—big things and little things. He constantly felt the need to check back with his partners over and over again to be certain he was working on the correct assignments and was doing them properly. "Was the Allen account up to date? Did the Johnsons need a letter? Were we changing the Samuelson's will?" Too many details, too many accounts. His nervousness was obvious. He began wringing his hands and pacing. He said he had a tape recording circling in his head with negative thoughts and feelings that wouldn't stop running. The vicious cycle of negativity couldn't be broken. He also began to make mistakes. It was after a year or two of this behavior that his partner told him to take time off and consult his doctor.

When Albert appeared at his family doctor's office his coat and tie were neat and tidy, but his furrowed brow and down-turned mouth belied his tense and worried nature. His doctor easily recognized his anxiety and also thought he was depressed. He prescribed an antidepressant and sent him to see a psychiatrist. The psychiatrist was impressed with both his anxiety and depression and added another medication. After a few weeks, Albert was worse rather than better. He rated his anxiety as a 9 or 10 on a 10-point scale and gave his depression a similar score. Although he wanted to return, there was no way he could go back to work. His psychiatrist responded that his illness was serious enough that he should try ECT. The doctor felt confident that this approach would work and he would experience a significant improvement after five treatments.

Why would ECT be tried on someone with HD? Electroshock treatment, later referred to as electroconvulsive therapy (ECT), was first introduced for psychiatric diseases in Italy, in the late 1930s. It became commonly used especially for severe depression in the United States in the 1940s and 1950s. At first, patients were actually given an induced seizure that sometimes led to injury or bone fracture. Later, short-acting sedatives and muscle paralytic agents were used to eliminate injury from a seizure. Side effects then became surprisingly minimal, except for varying degrees of memory loss. Even this problem was reduced when the stimulating electrode was placed on only one side of the head rather than both sides (bitemporal) (Figure 13.1). Improvement in deep depression unresponsive to medication was often impressive. The use of ECT has always made the public skeptical, if not

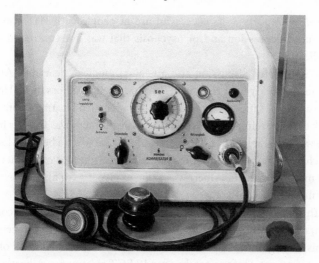

Figure 13.1 ▓ Electroconvulsive therapy (ECT) machine similar to that used on Albert Sullivan.

outright uncomfortable, which was underscored and heightened by the description of ECT in Ken Kesey's novel *One Flew Over the Cuckoo's Nest*. At least six films depicting ECT have received Academy Awards or nominations (*One Flew Over the Cuckoo's Nest*, with Jack Nicholson; *A Beautiful Mind*, with Russell Crowe; *Changeling*, with Angelina Jolie; *Revolutionary Road*; *Requiem for a Dream*; and *Frances*—the story of Frances Farmer, who was at Western State Hospital). In all of these Hollywood presentations ECT is depicted in an exaggerated or even cruel manner. A history of being treated with ECT essentially resulted in Thomas Eagleton stepping down from the national vice-presidential race in 1972, amid a torrent of negative publicity.

On the other hand, Kitty Dukakis, wife of the democratic presidential candidate in 1988, wrote a revealing memoir describing the highly successful treatment of her serious depression with ECT. In a TED talk, in 2001, Dr. Sherman Nuland, the highly regarded author of several popular medical books for the general public, dramatically related how ECT had literally saved his life. There has been no systematic study of using ECT in the treatment of HD, but there are several anecdotal reports of its successful use in people with HD who had advanced depression and/or psychosis that was not controlled with medication.[1]

With careful discussion and a general medical clearance, Albert began his weekly ECT treatments in another clinic across town. He felt confused and fatigued for several hours after each treatment, but was back to his baseline the following day. The problem was that his baseline was miserable. After the five treatments, he was no better. Albert's psychiatrist responded that they should press on and recommended five more treatments. Albert was game to give it a try and underwent five more weeks of ECT.

This was not easy. Slowly recovering from the post-ECT confusion, Albert then had to wonder if he could discern any improvement in his feelings and then would start to worry with anticipation of the next treatment. Unfortunately, after 10 ECT treatments, Albert's anxiety and depression continued, without abatement. His psychiatrist allowed that he was a "tough case," but that they should not stop now. The doctor recommended five more treatments, this time with bilateral stimulation. The previous 10 treatments had just used a single stimulator on one side of his head. Now the shocks would be given simultaneously on both sides. Albert was a bit reluctant, but felt like Macbeth: he had "stepped in so far" that there was no way to return, and he might as well plunge forward. He was fortunate to have a wife who was a calm and steady force in their marriage.

Fifteen ECT treatments did Albert no good. In fact, he was worse. Not only did his anxiety and depression remain untouched, but he was now more confused and lost several points on his cognitive test scores. He and his wife distinctly remember his psychiatrist concluding, "You are the worst case I have ever had!" Perhaps the doctor had just meant this as an off-the-cuff observation, to emphasize how hard his depression had been to treat, but Albert took this statement as a devastating blow. It made his depression worse. In any event, this gloomy physician suddenly moved to a new city and Albert presented his untreatable self to a new psychiatrist.

His new doctor was a woman who seemed empathetic, concerned, and willing to try new approaches. She switched him to a different medication. She also commented that she noticed subtle jerking of his hands and twitching of his body that were out of the ordinary. She said that his whole presentation reminded her of Huntington disease, but this seemed unlikely because of his age and lack of a family history (both his parents had lived to age 92). Nevertheless, she decided to send him to a neurologist for a second opinion. The potential diagnosis of Huntington disease struck Albert and his wife as coming out of nowhere and didn't make much sense, but they continued on to the next physician.

The neurologist agreed that HD was possible, but unlikely. However, she explained that the genetic blood test for HD should settle the issue and off Albert went to the lab. Lo and behold, the genetic test result returned "abnormal." The CAG repeat expansion was 38, lower than usually seen in most persons with HD, but definitely abnormal (see a more detailed discussion in the Appendix).

What an unexpected chain of events. After four doctors, Albert now had a new and totally unexpected diagnosis: Huntington disease. He and his wife were given complete detailed genetic counseling. They now realized that, in addition to his own diagnosis, their two adult children were also at 50% risk for HD. Meanwhile, there still remained the problem of his poorly treated anxiety and depression. These distressing symptoms could be coming from a multitude of causes, but it seemed likely that HD was a contributing factor. Still, he had not responded to a battery of medications, nor to ECT. In fact, the ECT made him worse.

As we have seen, depression is common in HD, occurring in at least half the patients sometime during the course of the disease. It is often ascribed to a somber realization that one has the disease. This was not the case with Albert, since his depression preceded any inkling that he had HD. His extreme anxiety and depression could have been coincidental and unrelated to his HD. More likely, these symptoms were actually a manifestation of the disease disrupting parts of the brain involved with emotions and feelings.

After nearly six months of no improvement on antidepressants, Albert's new psychiatrist said, "Let's try TMS." Of course, Albert and his wife asked, "What is TMS?" TMS stands for transcranial magnetic stimulation (Figure 13.2), and although this technique has some similarity to ECT, it uses a series of magnetic impulses, rather than an electric shock to the brain, during which the patient feels little or nothing. A variety of devices are placed over a particular area of the head and for 15 to 20 minutes the magnetic impulses are directed toward a specific region of the brain.

This description was good enough for Albert. He was desperate and willing to try anything that had a low chance of harm.

He started daily TMS treatments subsequently followed by treatments once a week. Albert, his wife, and his psychiatrist all agreed that within a few weeks the results were positive and clearly beneficial. Both the anxiety and depression were improved. On a daily basis he scored these two symptoms as 2–3 or 4–5 out of 10, rather than the

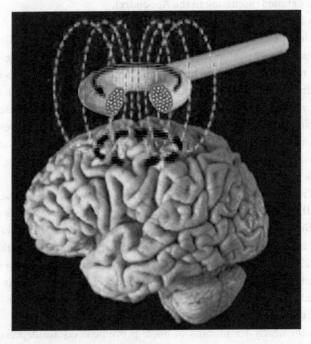

Figure 13.2 ■ Artist's representation of transcranial magnetic stimulation (TMS) (from Wikipedia), which was performed on Albert Sullivan after failure of ECT treatments.

previous 9 or 10. He was sleeping better. He was going for walks with his wife. He had returned to singing in the church choir. The vicious cycle had been broken. Although there have been only a few small clinical studies of TMS treatments in HD, it is clear that Albert's "trial of one" had shown improvement. Although Albert is not back to normal, he is improved and stabilized. He and his wife feel they have been given more quality time, even a new lease on life. It is no small thing to have the oppressive weight of chronic depression even partially relieved.

Of course, the TMS did not halt the progression of HD. A year later, Albert's anxiety and depression returned, with more disabling movements. The TMS was no longer helpful and Albert eventually entered hospice care at home.

Reference

1. Cusin C, Franco FB, Fernandez-Robles C, DuBois CM, Welch CA. Rapid improvement of depression and psychotic symptoms in Huntington's disease: a retrospective chart review of seven patients treated with electroconvulsive therapy. *General Hospital Psychiatry,* 35(6):678.e3–5, 2013.

14

"I Don't Agree"

"I don't think I have Huntington's but I want your opinion. I saw you 18 years ago when I was 50 and you said I showed no signs of it. My father died of Huntington's in his 60s but had his first signs of it in his 40s or 50s. My brother died with Huntington's in his 50s and showed his first signs in his 40s. I am retired but I still play squash. My friend says my coordination isn't as good as it used to be and he's worried about my health. I am 68 and I think I am still in pretty good shape. I think it is just normal aging. I don't think I have this disease. I thought you didn't get it after age 60. I want your opinion."

That was Mr. Z's statement as he sat in our clinic next to his wife. He was a short, slightly balding gentleman neatly attired in a dress shirt and sports coat. I had indeed seen him 18 years before and his examination had been entirely normal. Now he had obvious chorea. His speech was hesitant and jerky, he could not sit still in his chair.

He bobbed and weaved like a middleweight boxer. He even had a little twitch of his nose and cheek that fired off every minute or two. His movements were not severe, but perfectly noticeable to all the clinic staff. The strategy would be to gently inform him of this new development, trying not to be too negative or depressing.

I began by telling him that it was true that most persons with HD developed symptoms before age 60. However a few, perhaps 10%, develop their first signs of the disease after the age of 60. It was good news that his exam had been normal at 50 but even at 68 he was still at risk for the disease. Mr. Z said he wanted another exam to see what I thought now. I spent about 15 or 20 minutes checking his gait, eye movements, coordination and reflexes.

"Well, what do you think? I'm ok, right?"

"In general you are ok, but your coordination is a bit off. I think you have some problems in that regard that were not there 18 years ago."

"That doesn't make sense. I don't agree. I think my coordination is fine." He turned to his wife and asked, "What do you think?"

With no hint of any kind about what she might really think she said, "Don't ask me. Ask the doctor."

"Well I don't agree. I think I am just fine. Isn't there some kind of more accurate test you can do?"

"Yes, there is a fairly simple and highly accurate DNA-based genetic blood test that can tell us whether you have inherited the genetic changes associated with HD or not."

The genetic counselor and I then spent some time explaining the ins and outs of genetic testing for HD.

Finally, Mr. Z said, "I don't think I want that test right now. I feel fine. Can I think it over and come back if I change my mind?"

"Yes, certainly. There is no hurry, take your time."

Mr. Z left the clinic a little puzzled and not entirely satisfied with the interaction. He represented a common observation in patients with HD. He had obvious involuntary movements that were producing impaired coordination, but he was completely unaware of them. It used to be called "denial." That term did not seem quite right because there is no conscious denial of the movements; the person truly is unaware. The better phrase that is now used is "lack of awareness." (The official neurological term for this deficit is *anosognosia*, where *anosia* literally means "no knowledge.") This lack of awareness comes in many flavors, most famously demonstrated by Oliver Sacks' patient who mistook his wife for his hat.[1] Somehow the jumps, twists and turns that are obvious to us do not register on the patient's visual or sensory consciousness. It is a major problem for caretakers because the patient thinks there is no problem. They assume they are just as physically competent as ever. It is like a two-year-old running into the street unaware of the danger posed by traffic. Or like a four-year-old who can't swim, jumping into a pool.

We heard nothing more from Mr. Z until eight months later, when he returned to clinic. He had changed his mind about the testing. He decided he wanted to convince his family, his friends, his doctors and probably especially himself that he did not have HD. He was quite certain the test result would be normal. After again carefully reviewing the implications of genetic testing and indicating that I expected the test to show the DNA change associated with HD, he had his blood drawn and returned two weeks later. The test was positive. He indeed had the mutation related to HD. He shook his head in disbelief. He said it just made no sense to him. He felt fine. I pointed out that his number of 41 CAG repeats in the DNA, although abnormal, was on the low side of abnormal. It was typical of persons who had late onset of symptoms and fit with his situation. He said he thought we should repeat the test. I responded that we rarely did that. The test is highly accurate and, in fact, the result made sense and was what I expected.

"I want to get a second opinion. Is that ok with you?"

"Yes, that is fine. I have no problem with that."

"What about the Mayo Clinic? Isn't that a good place to go for a second opinion?"

"Yes, that would be fine."

It was easy to understand Mr. Z's disbelief about his diagnosis. He really did feel "fine" and could not imagine there was anything seriously wrong. He felt trapped by other people maneuvering him into places he didn't want to go.

Our records were sent to the Mayo Clinic and three or four months later I received a copy of the letter Mayo sent to Mr. Z. It said that he had some mild involuntary movements. They repeated the blood test and found 41 CAG repeats. This confirmed the genetic diagnosis of HD.

Mr. Z was back in our clinic after receiving the letter.

"Well, I guess the blood test was accurate, but I feel fine. I think my coordination is just fine. What do you think now that you have seen me over the past year? Do you still think I have abnormal movements, or have you changed your mind?"

Of course his movements were still there. They varied from time to time. They were less obvious when he sat calmly and more prominent when he was talking or excited. I told him I had not changed my opinion.

"What about driving? Do you think I should be driving?"

"I think you should not be driving. I think it would be safer for you and the people around you if you relied on your wife to be your chauffeur or used buses and taxis."

"Well, I think my driving is just fine. Isn't there some kind of test I can take to prove it?"

"You can take a driver's test from the state licensing office. If you flunk it you lose your license. The rehabilitation department in our hospital also has a consultant who gives detailed driver's exams. It's expensive and not always covered by insurance."

"I want to take that second kind of test," he answered.

Surprisingly, with a detailed letter justifying the need, his insurance company agreed to cover the cost.

A few weeks later I received the results of the evaluation. The conclusion: this man should not be driving. His fine motor coordination and visual spatial abilities are poor.

Mr. Z did not fight it. He gave a big sigh and stopped driving. He and his wife are grappling with his new diagnosis and coping quite well. He likes to read and take long walks. He still thinks his coordination is far better than it is, but he is being cautious and remaining safe. Lack of awareness has the advantage of allowing a person not to be forced to recognize their disability every minute of the day.

■ ■ ■

Betty Crowley was also blissfully unaware of her disease. She would come to the clinic with her husband, fortunately, a thoughtful, patient caretaker. Betty had thin blonde hair that stuck out in all directions and a small, bird-like face with sharp blue eyes. Everything was good with Betty. No problems. No difficulties. A-OK. She paid close attention to questions but never spoke in sentences. In fact, her limited vocabulary consisted almost exclusively of two words: *yip* and *nope*.

"Is everything ok today?"

"Yip."

"Are you taking your medicines?"

"Yip."

"Any problems?"

"Nope."

"Can we help you with anything?"

"Nope."

Each "yip" and "nope" was said quickly and sharply, with a sudden little jerk of her head and a jump of her body. Her husband would just smile and shake his head with each of her responses. She reminded me of the so-called Jumping Frenchmen of Maine. This was a small group of French Canadians, in the first part of the 20th century, who worked in the forests and lumber mills of Maine and New Brunswick. The men and a few women were notorious for having a strange habit of giving a sudden jump and vocalization whenever surprised or startled. Their coworkers made a practical joke out of suddenly clapping or yelling and causing them to jump and shout. Several different neurologists studied them, trying to determine if they had a brain disorder like Tourette's syndrome. The final conclusion was that it probably represented a cultural and psychological affliction, not a genuine brain disease. The Jumping Frenchmen did not have a progressive disease. Betty did. Last time I saw her she could still walk but was almost mute. Very few "yips" and "nopes."

■ ■ ■

Gordon Thomas was also a striking example of lack of awareness. He was a tall, muscular young man who could have been a linebacker.

In fact, he did play high school football. Now he lived by himself in a one-room apartment and spent his time aimlessly wandering around his small town. His mother had died of HD, and he was surviving on Social Security Disability. He had a court-appointed caretaker who lived in the same building. The caretaker cooked his meals, kept track of his bank account, and tried to keep him out of trouble.

In the clinic Gordon's attitude was much like Betty Crowley's "everything was fine." He had no complaints. One day while I was interviewing him the room developed an aroma of urine. When he stood up it was clear he had wet his pants. His blue jeans had a huge dark stain. His caretaker said it happened often. Gordon, meanwhile, was completely unaware of his accident. His brain was disconnected from his bladder. Just as some HD patients can have disinhibited behavior (like Jenny in Chapter 11 and Carolyn in Chapter 12), others can have a disinhibited bladder. Our nurse provided him with a dry, thick, adult diaper and a supply for later. The same thing happened during his next clinic appointment and he remained unaware and unconcerned. We prescribed a medication to inhibit his bladder, but he didn't like pills and didn't take them.

Later we learned Gordon also had a strange attitude toward his bowel movements. He stored his underpants full of feces in a bureau drawer and his caretaker would only discover this when the smell became noticeable. Gordon sometimes smeared feces over the furniture, doors and windows in his apartment and the cleanup might take hours. He was unconcerned with the effect of this on others and became angry when told to stop. He was strong and his belligerence could be scary. His behavior seemed to be a strange and unfortunate combination of lack of awareness and disinhibition. Later in his disease course Gordon was admitted to a private hospital for pneumonia. After he recovered it was impossible for the hospital to transfer him elsewhere. No other place was willing to accept him because of his long record of past misbehavior. So there he stayed, medically healthy, for almost an incredible two years until he was finally moved to a nursing home. This might be the HD equivalent of the wealthy New York heiress who liked her hospital so much she remained there for 20 years.[2] Gordon didn't last that long, but I suspect he was a lot more trouble for the nurses.

Mr. Z, Betty, and Gordon were coping with their disease in their own unique ways as adults. Coping strategies may change when there is more time to establish a lifestyle, as we will see in the next chapter.

References

1. Sacks O. *The Man Who Mistook His Wife for His Hat.* Simon and Schuster, New York, 1970.
2. Dedman B, Newell PC. *Empty Mansions: The Mysterious Life of Hugette Clark and the Spending of a Great American Fortune.* Ballantine Books, New York, 2014.

The Greatest Generation and Productive Lifestyles

About 5–10% of persons with Huntington disease develop their first symptoms before the age of 20, and 1–2% develop symptoms before the age of 10. At the other end of the spectrum is 5–10% of the HD population who have late onset of symptoms. We previously saw Mr. Z, who was surprised to have his first symptoms develop after the age of 60 and was largely unaware of his disability.

Even older than Mr. Z was Mr. Jacobson, who was referred to our clinic at the Veterans Affairs (VA) Hospital when he was a still vigorous 79. He was born in the Midwest of parents who were immigrants from Sweden. Raised during the Depression, he joined the Army during World War II and was trained as a paratrooper. He jumped behind enemy lines and received a Purple Heart for a shrapnel wound in his leg. He was one of the real heroes of the "Greatest Generation." Following the war, Mr. Jacobson married, had a son and moved to the Pacific Northwest, where he had a long career of hard physical labor in the timber industry. He developed severe hearing loss and wore hearing aids in both ears for most of his later adult life. Happily transitioning into retirement in his mid-60s, he spent much of his time hunting and fishing in the beautiful green forests and lakes of Western Washington. In his mid-70s, he stumbled and fell while hunting and accidently discharged his rifle. No one was injured and the incident was written off as a trivial accident. In retrospect, this may not have been a simple accident. Later, on a routine visit to his family doctor at age 79, it was noticed that he was twitchy and jumpy and seemed to have movements he couldn't control. His wife volunteered that he was also clumsy using his tools at home and was not doing his usual meticulous household handiwork.

On meeting him in our clinic he was a large, broad-shouldered man with thick, strong hands. He was neatly dressed in a tan sports coat and brown necktie. He came from an era when one dressed up for a doctor's appointment. He indeed had trouble sitting still and clearly had mild but definite twitches of the face and arms. Even with his hearing aids he had trouble following conversation. His aids had that troublesome characteristic of suddenly giving off a high-pitched noise. He would remove one, swear under his breath, tap it in his hand, and replace it. His speech pattern had the long drawn-out monotone common in people with deafness. His speech was also staccato and interrupted by short grunts caused by involuntary contractions of his diaphragm. He had no family history of HD or any other neurological disease. However, his wife mentioned that her father-in-law was fidgety and had trouble sitting still the last few years of his life. That man died of cancer in his 80s. Because Mr. Jacobson's involuntary movements were causing some problems and he and his doctor wanted some explanation, and because he had a son, we agreed to proceed with genetic testing. His genetic test was positive, with 39 CAG repeats. This is a relatively small CAG expansion, but the result is recognized to be abnormal and exactly the expansion size most commonly seen in later onset of the disease.

We followed Mr. Jacobsen yearly for the next decade. He continued to drive even though we advised against it. His wife was very supportive and quietly monitored him carefully, basically keeping him out of trouble. His chorea slowly became more noticeable but never seemed to be a major problem and required no treatment. He would usually point to his squeaking hearing aids and say, "These damn things are my biggest problem, not that other little disease you said I have. What's its name?"

Mr. Jacobson died quietly of a heart attack at age 89. He was a genuine old-fashioned, blue-collar gentleman and we always enjoyed his visits to the clinic. He was, however, not the oldest person I have seen with HD. That distinction goes to Mr. G, whom I first met at age 91. A successful retired businessman, his family thought he had been "a little nervous and fidgety" for 15 or 20 years, but nothing concerning. He was getting along quite well in his retirement home. When he was 90, his family doctor decided he had too many movements and sent him to a neurologist. She thought it was most unlikely he would have HD because of his age and the apparent lack of anyone in his family with HD, but ordered the genetic test "just to be complete." To everyone's surprise, his test was positive, with 39 CAG repeats. Now his four adult children and multiple grandchildren were suddenly at risk for HD. Mr. G was also a veteran, having spent World War II as a corpsman in a naval hospital. If one could choose the type of HD he or she would develop, this would be it: late onset and relatively mild symptoms compatible with a long and productive life, like that experienced by Mr. Jacobsen and Mr. G.

In the VA Medical Centers in Seattle and Tacoma I have seen more than 100 veterans who carried the mutation for HD. They have participated in all our country's wars over the past 75 years. They have served their country on the front lines in Europe and in the island campaigns in the South Pacific and in Korea, during the Tet Offensive in Vietnam, and in the recent protracted fighting in Iraq and Afghanistan. I have seen men and women whose HD has been compounded by posttraumatic stress disorder (PTSD) and repeated blast injuries.

It is also worth pausing to recognize the multitude of persons having the mutation for HD who have led successful, productive and creative lives both before developing symptoms of HD and after symptoms have started. Woody Guthrie is, of course, the role model for this category. A short list of individuals I have seen who reflect this positive perspective includes the following:

- A nuclear chemist with a degree from MIT whose career was devoted to medical diagnostic testing
- A university professor of geology
- A physician board certified in internal medicine who specialized in allergy and immunology
- A lovely woman who was a professional model and piano teacher
- A commercial airline pilot who had previously flown in the Air Force
- A firefighter with a long career protecting Seattle-Tacoma International Airport
- Numerous popular and committed elementary and high school teachers who have taught hundreds of children
- A Boeing aerospace engineer who worked on the development of the 747
- A Phi Beta Kappa university graduate who became an attorney and a partner in his law firm
- A professional artist whose budding career was cut short by the disease
- A Lutheran minister who taught theology and traveled extensively as a tour guide in Europe and the Holy Land
- A woman who had her own interior-design consulting business
- An accomplished woodworker who created beautiful cabinets and furniture
- A molecular neuroscientist doing outstanding research on his own disease

- An architect who helped design dozens of homes and buildings that provide pleasant working and living spaces to thousands of people

Having the genetic mutation for HD can be compatible with a productive and joyful life. In fact, there are thousands of persons presently alive with the HD mutation carrying on daily lives of every sort, largely unaware of their genetic makeup. From a genetic perspective, we all have genes with a variety of mutations putting us at risk for unexpected diseases. This knowledge can be reassuring or distressing, depending on one's point of view.

16

Princess in Pink

As mentioned earlier, at the other end of the HD spectrum are children who develop symptoms before age 10. Little Bobbi was excited to start kindergarten and begin her journey through elementary school. She was a happy kid who enjoyed kickball and coloring with crayons. Her favorite color was pink. She moved easily through school, learning to read and write. She was a favorite of her teachers. In third grade her family noticed that her right foot was turning in and kickball was no longer so easy. It seemed a trivial concern. However, at the parent–teacher conference in fourth grade the news was not so good. Physically she could no longer keep up with the other children on the playground. Academically she was not only falling behind her peers, but her writing and math skills were worse than what she had accomplished in third grade. The teacher strongly advised getting a doctor's advice.

Bobbi's father and grandmother were very worried. They explained the situation to her pediatrician. Bobbi's mother had died at age 34 with Huntington's disease and her mother, Bobbi's grandmother, had died at age 32 of the same disease. The family knew about developing HD at a young age (known as juvenile HD). They were also aware that, for unknown reasons, almost all children with HD inherited the disease from their father, not their mother. Nevertheless, the pediatrician was concerned and sent Bobbi to a pediatric neurologist at Seattle Children's Hospital.

The neurologist found that Bobbi was friendly and tried hard to cooperate but was clumsy, slow to move and had stiffness in her legs. She had no involuntary movements. She had short, brown hair, was very shy and clung tightly to her grandmother's arm. Like most children, she had no interest in being in a doctor's office. Her large, darting eyes and rare, quick smile indicated close attention to the conversation and action swirling around her. The genetic counselor discovered that Bobbi's mother had been evaluated in her late 20s in the University of Washington HD Clinic. Her mother's genetic test demonstrated the abnormality and she even had a remarkably high number of 62 CAG repeats in the *HTT* gene. This large number of unstable repeats, combined with the very young ages at death of Bobbi's mother and grandmother, were disturbingly ominous for predicting childhood onset of the disease in Bobbi.

Juvenile HD is uncommon but well recognized. About 10% of all people with HD have onset of symptoms before the age of 20, and about 2% have onset of symptoms before age 10. The fidgety chorea movements that occur in adults are usually not seen in children. This absence of chorea makes it more difficult to identify the early symptoms of the disease. The first sign is often a decline in schoolwork in a student who was previously doing very well. Increasing clumsiness on the playground is also common, as well as stiffness of the arms and legs and unsteady walking with frequent falls. Epileptic seizures occur in many of the children who have onset before the age of 10. Such seizures are quite uncommon in adults. Progressive deterioration in juvenile HD is more rapid than in adults and lifespan from onset of symptoms is frequently only about eight years. Childhood onset of HD is closely correlated with an unusually large number of CAG repeats (expansion). In juvenile HD the CAG expansion is usually greater than 60 and frequently much higher. The largest repeat expansion we have ever seen in our clinic was 165, which is extraordinarily high. This occurred in a cute little boy who had onset of clumsiness at about age three and died shortly after his sixth birthday.

It is a difficult choice to decide whether or not to test a child who is at risk for a serious genetic disease for which there is no cure and no prevention. This is especially tricky for a disease which usually has an adult onset. The general consensus is not to test such children if they have no symptoms. This would prevent them from being labeled as having a disease that was presently causing them no problems and might not manifest for several more decades. Most parents could not refrain from thinking about the child's abnormal test result every time the child had an emotional, social or physical problem (and what child doesn't?). Would the child be overprotected? Would teachers or other family members be told of the test result? Should the child be told? Would there be a so-called self-fulfilling prophecy of cascading problems attributed, perhaps wrongly, to HD? This is the labeling to be avoided.

The equation changes if the child has symptoms suspicious of the disease. In that case, there may be a medical treatment for some of the symptoms, if not the disease itself, and special help and accommodations available in school. Also, if the genetic test does not show the mutation related to HD, then that genetic disease is eliminated as a diagnosis and the family and physicians can focus their attention on other possible causes of the symptoms.

After careful consideration and counseling, the family and the doctors decided to proceed with genetic testing. Bobbi's test showed the mutation. She had 82 CAG repeats, even higher than her mother's test and fully compatible with the childhood onset of HD. Bobbi had juvenile HD.

This was a terrible blow to her family. The mother had died at an early age with HD and now her 10-year-old daughter was already showing signs. While the adults in the family could express their sadness, it was hard to tell what was going through the Bobbi's mind. She had heard many conversations about HD in her family long before coming to the clinic. She knew she was seeing doctors because of the concern she might have HD. She knew her genetic test was positive. She was quiet, shy and talked little about her concerns. She returned to school. Her teachers and friends gathered around and were very supportive. She had special classes and regular sessions with physical therapists and psychological counselors. She continued to work hard and had a remarkable steadiness and equanimity. She never complained, but her clumsiness and slowness had become obvious. Her fifth-grade teacher, Miss Perry, decided to be proactive. She wanted to make Bobbi more comfortable in the classroom and educate her other students about Bobbi's disease and how to relate to persons with disabilities. Thus began the Princess Project.

The class discussed Huntington disease and created a booklet about Bobbi and her condition. The cover, of course, was pink and had a picture of Bobbi wearing a pink crown. The title was "Princess in Pink." The booklet was about 30 pages long and contained observations about Bobbi along with drawings of her activities that were created by her classmates (Figure 16.1) (reproduced with permission of Bobbi's teacher and grandmother). The pages went like this:

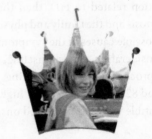

Figure 16.1 ■ The fifth-grade classmates of Bobbi, who had juvenile Huntington disease, produced this booklet describing their 11-year-old friend. (Photo with permission of guardian and teacher.)

This is a book about our classmate Bobbi and her life with Huntington's disease. Our life changed in the first day of fifth grade when we met our new classmate Bobbi. We learned about the changes that were happening to her body because of the disease. We decided to write a book about her in the hopes of finding a cure.

Princess in Pink: A little girl who looked pretty in pink it doesn't matter where it is maybe in her hair. She likes hot pink and other colors too. Her nickname should be pinky: you brighten my life Pinky. She is like a pink highlighter but a pink life lighter. If she could I bet she would either have a pink pony or a pink kitty. She probably has a ton of pink carnations in her house. I wonder what the heart of pinky's life looks like. She is bright pink inside and out. She is like the princess of pink. What would life be like when you're sick? WHAT WOULD LIFE BE LIKE HAVING HUNTINGTON'S DISEASE?

The Disease: Bobbi has inherited Huntington's disease (HD) from her mother. Her mother passed away two years ago. Bobbi was diagnosed shortly after her mother's death. This disease has affected people from 2 through 81. Anyone whose mom or dad has the disease has a 50/50 chance of getting it. HD can last from 10-25 years before you pass on from it. Here are some of the symptoms (there are *'s by the ones that Bobbi has developed in 2002–2003): *Personality changes, depression, *mood swings, *unsteady balance, wild movements, *slurred speech, *impaired judgment, *difficulty in swallowing, acting intoxicated. Bobbi has developed a lot of these symptoms, but not all of them.

Recess: Bobbi loves recess. She mainly plays "Tag, you're it." When we are out at recess, we play tag with Bobbi. Once she taps you, she runs to the grass and yells, "Base." Then she giggles her adorable little giggle that brightens your day. She also likes to play tetherball and soccer, but she will continue to play tag while she waits in line. Bobbi sometimes plays on the monkey bars too. She will hang on the bar for two seconds, and then let go. She NEVER plays with the boys, only the girls.

Animals: Bobbi loves animals. Her favorite animal is a pony. She also loves cats and dogs. Once she was even trying to buy a pony on eBay. She goes on search engines and looks at different animals. She has a kitty purse that she carries around everywhere. She always draws pictures of her favorite animals.

Smiling: Bobbi is so funny! She makes everyone smile, especially when you tickle her belly. She laughs so hard you can't help laughing with her.

School: Bobbi likes all of her friends at school. She also likes to play on the computer. She looks at animals, plays games, and tries to buy things on eBay. It is funny when you sit by Bobbi on the computer. She will tap your arm until you look at what she is doing. Bobbi loves to play with her friends at school and write letters to them. Sometimes she gets gifts from her "Secret Pal," which is Miss Perry. Miss Perry loves to give her fun stuff that Bobbi loves.

Food: Bobbi loves school food. She always gets a cheeseburger, if that is on the menu. She also loves hot dogs and chicken burgers. Miss Perry doesn't even have to wait for Bobbi, if she is late. She can just order for her. Bobbi also loves applesauce and ketchup.

Clothes: Bobbi always wears pink.

Make-up: Bobbi loves make-up. She always brings her lip-gloss to school. She probably wants to look her best for the boys. She puts it on like a princess. She has so many flavors that she has a different lip-gloss everyday. Of course if it doesn't smell good, she doesn't use it.

Strong (Figure 16.2): Bobbi is super strong when she wants to be. When she tells you that she is taking you to jail, she won't let go until she wants to. She can run really fast too. In P.E., we have a tug of war contest, and she was a real challenge. You would never expect something like that from her because she is so tiny.

Backpack: Bobbi always has tons of stuff on her desk. She has about five different water bottles, and she brings a different one everyday. She even has a headset that makes her voice louder like a microphone. Bobbi has about 10 million pencils. When we pack her up, at the end of the day, she has to put every single thing into her backpack. If you forget something she will scold you! Everyone knows not to mess with Bobbi when it comes to her backpack.

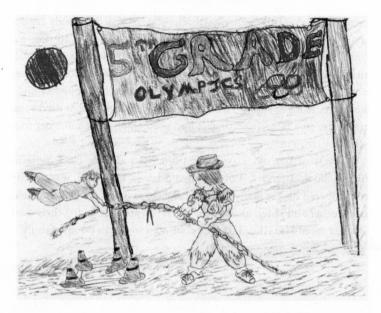

Figure 16.2 ■ A classmate of Bobbi drew this picture of her as a strong Olympic champion. (With permission of guardian and teacher.)

Now that you have read about Bobbi, you can see why she is so special to us. She is a wonderful and cheerful friend to everyone she meets. No matter what happens to Bobbi in the future, she will always be with us.

Miss Perry's approach was perfect. Bobbi continued to feel comfortable in school and her classmates responded to her in very positive and compassionate ways. It was a learning experience for everyone, including the adults.

As expected, Bobbi's disease was slowly but relentlessly progressive. She developed seizures that were successfully treated with anticonvulsant medication. She continued with three more years of school, but staying in the classroom became more and more challenging and her attendance waned. By age 13 she could no longer walk and required a wheelchair. She began to lose weight even though her appetite remained good. This "hypermetabolic" state in which the body cannot maintain weight is common in HD. We once cared for a 16-year-old boy with juvenile HD who lost weight even when taking in 10,000 calories a day. At age 15, Bobbi required a feeding tube. It became harder and harder for her to communicate. She eventually stopped talking, but never lost her smile. Tired and emaciated, little Bobbi died soon thereafter in a hospice setting. It had been eight years since her foot started to turn in.

Several of her old classmates from Miss Perry's class, now in high school, attended Bobbi's memorial service. She was fondly remembered by her many friends, teachers and family. This included her brother and sister, also at 50% risk, who are now facing their own worries about HD. The HD clock continues to tick in Bobbi's family.

PART III

Marriage, Family and Finances

An inability to form and sustain interpersonal relationships can be a fundamental problem for persons with HD. Thus, it should come as no surprise that HD can have major consequences on marriage and family life. The extreme variety of behaviors associated with HD can surprise and disorient family members. A spouse who knows nothing about HD can be confused and shocked by the unexpected personality changes in his or her partner. Children developing in the environment of a parent with HD may have no compass or guidebook to explain the perplexing behavior of a mother or father with the disease. The stress of the disease can sometimes disrupt a family beyond repair. At other times, the stress can be frustrating and damaging, but through bonds of remarkable, flexible strength the families survive intact. In some instances HD even seems to bring a family closer together.

Adoption is not rare in families with HD. This sometimes happens when a young woman who is already experiencing early symptoms of HD, including impulsivity and impaired judgment, finds herself pregnant and realizes she is incapable of raising a child. Three examples will be described of how adoption may play a role in the developing dynamics of this disease.

Huntington disease usually strikes individuals at midlife, a time when employment, earning a living wage and raising a family are expected and necessary. The symptoms of HD can wreak havoc on employment and managing finances, just when these skills are most important. This section will explore several ways in which persons with HD have struggled to maintain employment and to stay afloat in the world of finances.

17

For Better, for Worse

Because symptoms of HD typically develop in midlife, it is common for careers and marriages to begin in complete ignorance of the disease that may be hovering unrecognized in the future. This was the case with Ralph. He knew nothing about HD when he married Gloria. Gloria was a talented, vivacious redhead who owned an art gallery. When a distant relative was a diagnosed with HD and then Gloria's father started to behave oddly and was later diagnosed with HD, things began to change. The family signs were just too strong, and Gloria decided to have genetic testing: the genetic variant associated with HD was discovered. At first, no one thought she had symptoms, including her family and us, her clinicians.

As the years went by, Gloria slowly lost interest in her gallery. She lost interest in most things and spent her time sitting at home or going for long walks alone. She began to argue with Ralph, first about little things and then about almost everything. She accused him of hiding money from her. She accused him of having an affair. She wanted to move out. She wanted to end the marriage. She wanted to be by herself. They tried marriage counseling, but to no avail.

Gloria moved into a small apartment and continued to rant and complain about Ralph. Ralph sold their home and moved to another house. Blithely unaware of her growing disabilities, Gloria was unable to successfully shop for groceries or prepare her own meals. As she walked the streets her chorea and confusion and disheveled appearance made her an easy mark for abuse. Her siblings were finally able to move her into a retirement home that included assisted living. Now her independence was gone. She was safe, but often falling, and was argumentative with the staff. She began calling Ralph every day, pleading with him to come back. It was too late. He had moved on, and in any event, she needed full-time assisted living. The marriage had broken long ago, mostly as a result of HD.

■ ■ ■

Beth and Ken had a different relationship. Ken managed a grocery store, and Beth was a middle school teacher. They gardened together and were heavily involved with Boy Scouts. Ken had been a Boy Scout and Beth a Girl Scout and they now directed three different Scout troops. They loved it and it kept them very busy. Ken's father had died of HD and his brother had developed the disease a few years earlier. As Ken, too, developed symptoms, he made mistakes in the store and lost interest in his job. He had to retire but puttered around home while Beth continued to teach. Although they had to cut back to mentoring one Scout troop, Beth was able to remain involved. Ken quietly withdrew into a world of inactivity. The living room couch became his home. Beth smiled and shrugged her shoulders with a "that's the way it is" attitude. She was able to stay involved with a social life of her own.

■ ■ ■

Margaret tried to hold her family together against great odds. A few years after their marriage, her husband developed symptoms of HD, which he inherited from his father. She worked tirelessly, maintaining her home while her husband still lived with her. In addition to all the usual household tasks, she had to keep track of his medication and deal with his confusion and wandering. He eventually moved to an assisted living facility, where he died two years later. In spite of all this, Margaret volunteered as an HD educator. She and our clinic social worker formed a team that tirelessly visited nursing homes and retirement homes that were caring for persons with HD. Margaret was active in the early days of the national HD association.

Margaret also had to think about her children. She had three daughters and a son who had grown into young adulthood. They married and had children. First the oldest daughter and then the youngest daughter developed HD. Although their personalities were delightful, the disease became obvious and distressing. Both had progressively worsening movements that were difficult to control. The oldest also developed such severe confusion and inattention that she had to be placed in a nursing home. And then Margaret's son was also found to have the mutation causing HD. The weight of all this was overwhelming—her father-in-law, her husband, her two daughters, and now her son. Plus all those grandchildren who were now at risk for the disease. Margaret could no longer face HD. She was overwhelmed by the burden of this disease. It is no secret that HD has a tremendous impact on family members without the disease, especially those who take on the role of caretakers. Caught in this dilemma, Margaret was unable to reach out to others for assistance. Unfortunately, her solution was to take a massive overdose of sleeping pills that ended her life.

■ ■ ■

The hereditary nature of HD is the genetic twist that makes the disease so much worse. Carol Carr could have related to Margaret's struggles if they had known each other. Carol lived in a suburb of Atlanta and married into a family with HD: her husband and daughter died with HD. Another son committed suicide when he learned his HD test was positive. She had two more sons who also developed HD, and she watched them slowly move through the accumulating unyielding symptoms. Finally, both sons were in a nursing home in the advanced stages of HD, unable to walk or talk. Carol Carr made news headlines in 2002 when she walked into the nursing home and shot and killed both her sons.[1] She waited calmly for the police to arrive and was arrested and jailed. She said she had been at her "wit's end." The county prosecutor decided to press charges and she was found guilty of "assisted suicide" (not homicide). Her sentence was for five years and she was released after 21 months in prison. Her fourth son, and only living child, said, "She acted out of love, not malice." She could no longer stand the tremendous burden HD had dropped on her family.

■ ■ ■

Ron Allen operated a large power saw in a lumber mill owned by the Weyerhaeuser timber company. He was a hard worker and had glowing comments in the personnel file. In his mid-40s, his work became sloppy and he made mistakes in simple arithmetic calculating the lengths of board to be cut. He made errors in his usually meticulous home repair jobs and lost interest in his family. He was forced to retire and was lucky to get a reasonable pension from his company. His wife gave up, sued for divorce, and requested complete child custody of their 8-year-old daughter and 10-year-old son. She had read about HD and feared its consequences. She thought Ron should have no further contact with his children. He asked to see them on weekends and to have them stay with him one weekend each month. We evaluated him in the clinic and found him to be a reasonable guy who was capable of caring for himself and seemed to understand the implications of his disease and his wife's concerns. I had to testify before a judge who needed background on HD and my opinion about Ron and his capabilities. It was a difficult medical and legal question. Ron had never shown evidence of abusing or neglecting his children and seemed to truly care for them. The judge decided to allow him the weekend visits for a trial period of six months and for these visits to be monitored by a specific social worker. It turned out to be a wise decision. The visits initially happened without incident. In fact, Ron and his kids even spent a weekend at Disneyland. However, as time passed, the social worker noticed that Ron seemed to be paying less attention to his children during the visits. They were also becoming interested in many other activities and probably were embarrassed by their father's disease. The visits ended in a mutually agreeable way, and Ron spent the last few years of his life in an assisted living facility.

■ ■ ■

The stories in this chapter show how difficult it is to hold a family together once HD intrudes. In the next story, in Chapter 18, we will see how George Wilson responded to his wife's slowly developing struggle with the disease.

Reference

1. Rimer S. A deadly disease destroys patients and families. *New York Times*, June 24, 2002.

18

In Sickness and in Health

Kay married George Wilson in her early 20s. He had a newly minted degree in engineering and they moved to Seattle for his new job with Boeing. He was especially talented with tools and drills of all kinds and was eventually part of the team that developed the B2 bomber. They had four children, and Kay used her degree in elementary education and early childhood development to be a full-time homemaker and mother. One of their children had difficult behavioral problems that fell somewhere along the attention deficit hyperactivity–autism spectrum. As this child grew older, Kay struggled with depression and anxiety, problems thought to be related to the stress of raising this difficult child.

During a visit to a psychiatrist to discuss the child's behavior, the doctor, as an aside, said that he noticed Kay had unusual persistent movements of her hands and fingers. Kay was now 40 years old. Kay and George were surprised at this observation but decided to follow the psychiatrist's suggestion that she seek a neurologist's opinion. The neurologist agreed with the psychiatrist. In fact, he said he was quite certain she had chorea and he was suspicious she might have Huntington disease. He ordered a brain MRI, which was normal. He asked if there could be any possible family history of such a disease and suggested she seek a second opinion at the University of Washington.

Kay said she could recall no one in her family who had any abnormal movements. George was more discerning. He said, "Remember that one time we met your father? He was a very nervous, jumpy guy."

Kay's parents had divorced when she was four years old. Kay's mother discovered that her husband had a habit of exposing himself to his little daughter and other neighbor children. She packed up and left and Kay never saw her father again. That is, never again, except for one brief time in her early 20s, shortly after her marriage to George. They didn't remember the circumstances and it was only a brief interaction. Nevertheless, George always remembered her father as a nervous, agitated person who couldn't sit still. Although they never saw him again, they heard from the family grapevine that years later he was arrested for child molestation and incarcerated in a prison in Arizona.

George started calling the Arizona prison system in an attempt to discover what had happened to Kay's father. He made numerous calls and was shunted from office to office and seemed to be getting nowhere. Incredibly, he eventually found someone who had access to her father's record, took pity on George and gave him the critical information he was seeking. Yes, her father had been in the Arizona prison system. Yes, he had been evaluated multiple times by the medical personnel. Yes, he had been given a diagnosis of possible Huntington's chorea. Yes, they would send copies of the prison medical records to Kay's doctor. Because of his neurological disability, Kay's father had been released from prison and placed in a half-way house, whose name and address, surprisingly, was given to Kay. Kay and George decided to visit Arizona and see for themselves whether her father looked like someone with HD according to the descriptions they had read. They called ahead and made arrangements to meet him in a Denny's restaurant. The meeting was brief, but her father, who was brought by a caretaker, was confused, slurred his speech, and had obvious involuntary movements that made it nearly impossible for him to even walk. One can only imagine how traumatic this visit must have been for Kay. Here she was, a thousand miles from home, sitting in a Denny's restaurant face-to-face with her father, of whom she had no recollection except being told he was a child abuser, and now realizing that this disheveled, disoriented old man had a terrible degenerative brain disease that had probably been passed directly to her.

Kay's return visit to our clinic simply confirmed what had already become clear. She had undergone a number of blood tests that excluded other rare possibilities. She had mild but definite movements and, coupled with the story of her father, it was clear that the family had HD and that she was affected. The diagnosis was confirmed by genetic testing.

Kay's recent bout of depression and anxiety, combined with the realization that she had abnormal movements, heralded the beginning of her symptomatic HD. In any event, she continued to see a psychiatrist and was put on a variety of antidepressants. Unfortunately, they were of little help and her behavior deteriorated. In addition to depression she developed confusion and agitation. She had trouble preparing meals and shopping for groceries. She became angry with George and with the children. She lost her temper and would hit them.

As Kay's behavior slowly spun out of control, George was desperate and searched for solutions. He attended a conference on HD and heard a specialist say that behavior problems were common in HD and notoriously resistant to treatment with medication. Having had personal experience with Kay, this was no news to George. The specialist then said that in his experience these behaviors in HD often improved with electroshock therapy, or electroconvulsive therapy (ECT). George had heard of ECT, but it never occurred to him that it could be beneficial in HD. He discussed this with Kay's psychiatrist, who was running out of drug alternatives. He decided to give ECT a try if George and Kay were willing. They were.

Kay had a two-day hospitalization for one ECT treatment. George says he will never forget the result. It was like magic. She was a new woman. She seemed to have a little trouble with short-term memory, but other than that she was "back to herself." Her depression was gone and she had no more temper tantrums. It was a real relief.

These encouraging results from a single treatment lasted several months, then Kay slipped back into a little depression and her antidepressant was restarted. After 8 months, the agitation and temper tantrums began to return, and by 10 months after the ECT she was back to her unhappy self. This led to a second ECT treatment, as an outpatient. Once again, the result was dramatic. Her behavioral problems disappeared and she was the "new woman" once again. And once again the pleasant results lasted about 10 months. After that period of time the nasty behavior returned. The psychiatrist thought it was time for a third ECT treatment, and George and Kay agreed. A sticking point appeared in that their insurance company refused to pay for the outpatient ECT whereas, strangely, they would pay for inpatient ECT. That meant the company would not spend $5,000 for an outpatient treatment but would spend $30,000 for the same treatment as an inpatient. Insurance-company decisions do not always make sense.

The third ECT treatment produced the same beneficial results. Once again, Kay was back on track. Life was good, but only for a period of months. Once again, 10 months later, Kay's behavior began to deteriorate. George began to worry about this yo-yo effect and wondered how many years they would face this roller coaster. Also, how many ECT treatments could she sustain? Her psychiatrist decided to try a different antidepressant, and put her on bupropion. Good fortune smiled on Kay and George once again: the new antidepressant was incredibly effective. George and the psychiatrist never knew whether it was the bupropion by itself or in combination with the three ECT treatments, but Kay's depression subsided and her temperament improved. Her behavior stabilized to a relatively good frame of mind. However, Kay was now 54, and her movements had become considerably worse. She was having trouble walking, dressing and using eating utensils. George decided to retire and care for his wife full-time. He found acreage in Wyoming and off they went, to start a new life together.

Kay's movements were becoming much more troublesome. She bumped into furniture when walking and would often fall going around corners. Her speech was more difficult to understand. George took her to see a neurologist in Denver who specialized in movement disorders, including HD. That neurologist suggested they try a new drug called Risperdal. The medication had been introduced to treat behavior problems in people with psychiatric problems, but it sometimes reduced involuntary movements. It seemed worth a try.

Once again, Kay had success trying a new therapy. The Risperdal had a calming effect on her movements and made life much easier. Eating was not as difficult as before and she was less likely to fall. George saw a dramatic improvement that lasted about two years. The disease, however, did not stop its relentless progression. Eventually, her walking became uncoordinated and tenuous enough to require a wheelchair. George was able to purchase a power chair, but Kay's hand movements were so uncoordinated that she could not operate the controls. George was able to find a system that allowed an attendant walking behind the chair to maneuver the controls.

The new power chair allowed George and Kay to continue attending church. However, when Kay was sitting in a chair, her movements would sometimes suddenly cause her entire body to surge forward and she would fall to the floor because she had no kind of restraint in the chair to hold her back. George was able to fashion a leather belt loosely around her chest that prevented these sudden movements from ejecting her out of her seat. He also discovered that whispering to her during the church service had a calming effect and the sudden jerks would temporarily disappear.

By this time, Kay's speech had almost entirely ceased. She could only occasionally utter one or two words. In spite of this problem, George was convinced that her mind was intact and that she was paying careful attention to her surroundings and conversations. Once, after church, a woman kindly told him that she was impressed with his ability to "bear this burden." George responded that, rather than a burden, he saw it as a blessing. The woman said, "Really? A blessing?" George said, "Let's ask Kay. Kay, is all this life with HD a burden or a blessing?" Kay smiled and blurted out, "Blessing!"

George continued to use little questions like this as a method of staying in contact with Kay, bringing pleasure into her life and checking for himself on her level of awareness and cognitive ability. One of his favorite questions was "Do you love me a little bit?" There would be no response from Kay. He would repeat the question and again, no response. Then he would say, "Do you love me a whole lot?" She would give a laugh and blurt out, "Whole lot!"

When he took Kay to the neurologist in Denver an X-ray study showed poor swallowing and a high risk of aspiration. Pneumonia and even sudden death from choking can occur with HD. Fortunately, her cough reflex was very good and she rarely aspirated food into her airway. Her weight, however, dropped down to 105 pounds (from over 120) because she was not able to take in enough calories. George switched to an entirely pureed diet including banana peanut butter sandwiches, her favorite. Her weight stabilized and actually increased. George and a hired caretaker spent a lot of time dropping food into a large blender. He also added a commercial thickener, discovering that he could purchase 25 pound boxes for $75. He also made a squeeze bottle with plastic tubing to provide her with adequate amounts of water, tipping her back to 45 degrees in a recliner and then squirting the water into her mouth. This system worked very well with almost no coughing. George the engineer was busily at work.

Moving Kay around the house and transferring her from bed to chair and chair to toilet became a major effort. Once again, George's engineering experience and fascination with gadgets came in handy. On one occasion when Kay tried to transfer from her chair to the toilet, the sudden lurch of her body slammed into the toilet and knocked it off its pedestal. George rigged up wooden "stabilizers" for the toilet that prevented this from happening. In addition, George developed and built an ingenious sling-and-pulley system that could move Kay from place to place by just pulling on a few small ropes. The system was attached to the ceiling, and George installed tracks on the ceiling as part of a transport apparatus. Eventually, with his pulley system he could pluck Kay out of a chair or her bed and move her from one room to another or into the bathroom along the ceiling tracks. This made toileting and bathing much easier. A neighbor commented that the system looked like a side of beef being moved around in a butcher shop and George agreed that that was about right. The important thing was that it worked!

In fact, it was while transferring Kay on her little ceiling railway that, one day, her body simply gave out and she quietly died. She was 64 years old and had had symptoms of HD for at least 24 years. This was at least five or six years longer than the usual symptomatic duration of HD, although not unheard of. George attributed this long time frame to the fact that Kay was a "tough person" and never gave up easily. It also had a lot to do with her attentive caregiver.

In looking back on his life dealing with HD, George would still emphasize that it was not a burden. Even in the advanced stage of the disease he recalls putting his arm around Kay and, with a whisper in her ear, asking her if she recalled this or that pleasant event in their past years together. She would often smile and whisper back, "Yes." George said he learned that marriage was more than just romantic love. It could also develop into service and sacrifice to the person you love. He said, "Kay was way ahead of me in knowing that, but I finally got it."

19

Money Problems

From time to time we all struggle with finances. Credit cards, checking accounts, savings, bills, mortgages, insurance premiums, and taxes—who doesn't get confused? The impaired judgment and lack of awareness that are so prevalent among people with HD make financial dealings a minefield for mistakes and miscalculations, which vary from the trivial and humorous to the devastating.

Andrew had been in the Army. He made it through basic training, was transferred to sprawling Fort Lewis, in Western Washington, and eventually ended up with a desk job as an office clerk in the base PX. After two or three years, his performance evaluations got worse and worse. He made frequent mistakes, was late for work, and seemed oblivious to his poor performance. He was also noticed to be stumbling, losing coordination, and developed slurred speech. Those observations eventually resulted in his being seen by a medical officer. On careful interrogation, it was discovered that his father had died of HD, and the doctor proceeded to genetic testing. After a long wait, Andrew's test returned positive, with an abnormal CAG expansion size in the gene for HD. This, of course, got him a one-way ticket directly out of the Army. It was a medical discharge, and he was considered both disabled and to be service connected for HD. This provided him with a monthly VA pension of a relatively small, but nonetheless useful, amount of cash and access to treatment.

Our clinic team first saw Andrew in the VA hospital when he was in his late 20s. He was homeless, moving from shelter to shelter, but mostly living on the street. He was tall, thin and gangly, wearing an unbuttoned checkered shirt and ripped blue jeans. He wore glasses with thick lenses and his hair was long, dark and uncombed with the musty aroma of someone who often sleeps outside in the rain. He walked slowly with a peculiar high step, looking like a heron with spectacles. Regardless of his appearance, he often smiled and had an air of "whatever" unconcern. The telltale involuntary twitches of his face, arms and body were readily apparent. We tried to convince him to find an apartment or a group home, but he would have none of it. He enjoyed the loose freedom with his buddies on the street.

We asked Andrew about his monthly VA pension. He smiled and said he kept it in his "bank." "Want to see my bank?" He proceeded to take off his untied shoe. Then he pulled off his dirty sock with a hole in the toe. Inside the sock was a wad of green bills. He laughed and said, "I got more of that in the other shoe. It's safe there."

The next time we saw Andrew he was not so happy. His glasses were broken and held together with duct tape. He said he was completely out of money. He had been arrested and put in jail for loitering, smoking pot, and being a general public nuisance. He made the mistake of telling his cellmate about his VA pension. His cellmate told him he had training as a "financial advisor." He told Andrew that if he turned over his pension money to him he would invest it and make Andrew a tidy profit. When they got out of jail, Andrew did exactly that. Over several months he turned over all his money to his ex-cellmate, who eventually disappeared, and Andrew never saw a tidy or any other kind of profit. He needed help. We teamed Andrew up with an experienced and savvy hospital social worker. She set up an account and became Andrew's rep payee. She was able to dole out Andrew's money to him on a regular basis and at least keep his finances safe. He didn't stop living on the street, continued to be occasionally abused by coarser vagrants, and was a frequent visitor to jail. He never understood how to manage his relatively meager income. Eventually, over several years, he entered a group home, lost the ability to swallow, and was placed in hospice. After about a 15-year downward course of symptomatic HD, Andrew died without family or friends, at age 38.

■ ■ ■

Eddie reminded me of Andrew. His father had died of HD, and Eddie had been unable to finish high school. His grades were poor, he showed no interest in the classwork, and he was absent from school more often than present. He tried odd jobs but they never worked out. He couldn't run a cash register, he couldn't cook a meal. When he washed dishes he broke more than he cleaned. He couldn't multitask, and he frequently did not show up for work. When we met him in the clinic he had rumpled blonde hair and was wearing dirty jeans with well-worn hiking boots. With a red fleece vest over a checkered shirt he looked like a typical Northwest teenager on a camping trip. His finger movements were clumsy and his handwriting was sketchy. He had no involuntary movements, but his genetic test showed the HD mutation, with a substantially large CAG repeat expansion.

Like Andrew, Eddie was a loner. He found a vacant lot 10 miles north of Seattle, pitched a tent, and set up "camp." There he lived for a number of months and was never bothered by the police. He found an old bicycle and would spend time cruising the neighborhood. Two or three days a week for a period of six months, he would ride his bicycle two miles to a bus stop and tie it to a tree. He and five or six other transients would be picked up by an old school bus and driven to Safeco Field, in downtown Seattle, the Mariners baseball stadium. On those days, he would while away the hours sweeping the trash out of the stands. He would push a broom and slowly collect peanut shells, popcorn, ketchup-stained paper napkins and mustard-coated hotdog wrappers. At the end of the afternoon he was given a $20 bill and bused back to his corner. Half-way through the summer he discovered that his bike had been stolen. He had no replacement and began walking the distance between his tent and the bus stop. It was not a big problem because he was never in a hurry. One day in September, he returned to his vacant lot only to discover that it was truly vacant; his tent had been stolen. His sleeping bag and a few cups and dishes were left behind. He now had no cover over his head and the Seattle rainy season was about to begin. Also, the Mariners baseball season was ending. He began wandering from one homeless center to another.

A concerned social worker in our clinic tried to find Eddie a room in a low-income apartment or halfway house. He wasn't interested. He would rather live on the street.

Eddie had many of the cognitive and behavioral hallmarks of HD: apathy, poor attention span, impaired judgment and inability to multitask. It was sad to see all these traits appearing in such a young person. His future looked grim.

■ ■ ■

Ward Wilson had a different problem. He was a retired insurance salesman. "Retired" because he mishandled several sales and couldn't keep his records straight. When we first met him, his mood could be summarized in one word: *manic*. He had wavy red hair and freckles and couldn't stop talking. His ever-flowing conversation was frequently interrupted with laughter and accompanied by hand gestures and finger-pointing. He resembled a W.C. Fields character: pompous, self-assured and deluded. He was on a tranquilizer, but it did not seem to help much. His wife informed us of their biggest problem. Unbeknownst to her, Ward wandered off one day and purchased a boat for $50,000. They only had $1,000 in a checking account and $15,000 in savings. She was now left with trying to return the boat and recoup their money. Meanwhile, he thought he had done nothing wrong and that "things would work out." He also told me he was thinking of applying to Harvard Law School and wondered what I thought about that. I told him I thought it was a very competitive institution and he would not make the cut. He disagreed and thought it was worth a try. I suggested he begin by taking some community college law courses. Ward's pressured speech, oblivious squandering of his family's savings, and inappropriate assumption he was ready for law school had all the characteristics of mania.

■ ■ ■

It is puzzling that mania and its opposite, apathy, can be symptoms of HD. What determines the appearance of one or the other is entirely unknown. Presumably, it reflects a variation in the molecular and biochemical pathology occurring in regions of the brain associated with emotional stimulus and excitement. In some people with HD the balance is tipped toward a profound lack of energy, causing the person to sit in front of the TV for hours at a time, with no comprehension of the program. In others there is a stimulation of physical and psychic energy, causing nearly non-stop pacing and walking, or a torrent of talking, or a rush of thoughts that even prevent sleep.

Woody Guthrie, American's best-known celebrity with HD, also seemed to have had genuine manic episodes. An exhibit of his life and work has shown that he produced an incredible, constant flow of poems, songs, comments and just words that consumed reams of paper and every scrap of writing material available to him. Woody never suffered from writer's block. He tried to write thousands of songs and was hugely successful with dozens of them. One cannot help thinking that HD must have contributed some important element driving his tremendous productivity and creativity.

Kay Redfield Jamison and many others have written extensively about the possible contribution of mania, depression, and bipolar syndrome to artistic creativity.[1] While the exact role of bipolar illness in creativity remains to be clarified, the manic episodes that accompany the condition frequently lead to terrible financial decisions, as demonstrated by Ward Wilson, whose mania was grounded in HD.

■ ■ ■

Leonard Reynolds was sent to us by his law firm and came with his very worried wife. He did not have much to say as she quietly laid out his story. Leonard was a highly educated, respected and successful accountant and tax lawyer who worked in a large, local law firm. Recently his partners discovered that he had been making numerous errors, confusing accounts and receiving an increasing series of complaints from clients. His records were a mess and full of mistakes. His firm realized this couldn't continue. Leonard would have to be released, essentially for incompetence. His colleagues were puzzled, indeed shocked, by this recent change in his abilities, but for the good of the firm, he had to go. When she found out, his wife was aghast. Despite her husband's occupation, she was the one who kept track of their personal checkbook and finances, so his money problems had never been apparent at home. This new behavior was completely uncharacteristic. She had known for many years that Leonard's mother had died with HD. Now she became concerned that he was developing the first symptoms. She brought this to the attention of the law firm which, until then, had never heard of HD. After some quick background reading they informed Leonard that they would put his separation proceedings on hold until he had been evaluated in our clinic.

Leonard appeared neatly dressed in coat and tie with a pleasant but somewhat vacuous and flat emotional tone. He admitted confusing the accounts but could give no explanation for why he had done it. He shook his head and said, "I guess I just made some mistakes." He seemed to be unsure of this reasoning but recognized he needed to say something. He said he was sorry, but showed no particular sign of anger or sadness. It was as if he understood he was supposed to express some regret, but really could not comprehend exactly what had happened or why his work had deteriorated and collapsed. His wife was very distressed and made it quite clear that, compared to his former self, this was a dramatic change. This new behavioral change was perfectly consistent with the impaired judgment and lack of empathy often seen in HD. After detailed genetic counseling we proceeded with genetic testing.

Leonard's test was positive. He had inherited the genetic mutation for HD from his mother. Now negotiations began with his employers.

It was my belief that HD was likely a major contributor to his recent fumbling financial activities. I explained this to his law firm in the context of what was known about HD and its effect on behavior, judgment and executive functions. After considerable deliberation, his firm rather thoughtfully, and kindly, decided not to fire him for incompetence, but let him have a medical retirement. In fact, to the great relief of his wife and family, Leonard was given a fine retirement party with accolades to his years of dedicated service. He became a quiet, slow-moving, apathetic homebody who produced no further problems and seemed to be content sitting at home reading the newspaper and daydreaming. Leonard was an apathetic contrast to Ward Wilson's mania, but their contrasting behaviors both resulted in financial mismanagement that seriously disrupted their families.

■ ■ ■

Bernie Burroughs also came to us with financial problems. He was 50 years old, and his father and uncle had died with HD. He never married, perhaps because of his family history of HD. He had lived for the past decade in the same house with his mother, who was a part-time nurse.

In spite of the HD in the family, Bernie had developed a successful career based on his engineering talent. He was good with his hands and loved tools, motors and fixing machines. He became an expert Porsche repair mechanic. This was his niche and he made the best of it. His Porsche repair shop in Seattle gained a national reputation. He hired several top auto mechanics, and broken motors were shipped to him for repair from all areas of the country. Bernie was Seattle's "Mr. Porsche."

Things began to go wrong two or three years before his visit to our clinic. Bernie began to lose the ability to use his tools and made costly repair mistakes. By the time he came to us, his mother said, this wonderful mechanical engineer had trouble using a screwdriver or even replacing a light bulb. Even worse, his financial situation had collapsed. He lost his employees and had to sell his business. Furthermore, he was left owing customers $50,000. It was also discovered that he had stopped paying taxes and owed the IRS more than $200,000. This personal debt was weighing heavily on his mind, and he could not stop focusing on it and obsessing about it.

Bernie came to our clinic wearing a rumpled, loose-fitting jacket that suggested some recent weight loss. He kept running his fingers through his hair, anxious and easily distracted. This was a man in serious distress. He had difficulty sitting still, with frequent adjustments of his position, sudden little head jerks and occasional twitches of his fingers—nothing severe, but clearly mild chorea. He was aware of his clumsiness and his difficulty with finances. He and his mother had come to the conclusion that he was probably developing his father's HD. He had already made up his mind that he wanted genetic testing. The test showed the mutation associated with HD and he accepted the results without much comment. He actually preferred concentrating on his multiple other medical problems, which included back pain, tooth pain, frequent headaches and insomnia. His conversations usually came back to his embarrassment over the debt to his customers and frustration with his inability to pay them back. Bernie's sense of personal ethics had been badly damaged and he saw no way of moving beyond it. Over the next several months, we saw him frequently and tried to systematically work on all his problems. He was given an antidepressant, a sleeping medication, and a drug for his involuntary movements that was also an antipsychotic.

Bernie turned out to have a tooth abscess, and his dentist was worried that removal would be difficult because of his uncontrolled movements. We decided to give him valium before the extraction to calm him and, fortunately, it worked like a charm. The tooth was out, his pain was gone, and we could scratch one problem off his list. We found a bankruptcy attorney who took on pro bono cases. This would be a helpful step in the right direction, but the appointment was a long way off. We learned that Bernie had a gun at home and strongly urged his mother and other family members to confiscate it. They said they would try, but knew he liked his gun and would be resistant. He had inherited a gun collection from his grandfather and was very attached to it.

Our clinic psychiatrist evaluated Bernie and we agreed that he was in an agitated depression. His persistent insomnia was a reflection of his obsessive worrying about his debt. Various sleep medicines were of some benefit, but we tried to keep the doses low because of our concern that he might take an overdose. When asked directly about suicide thoughts he denied them. There was a bed available on the hospital psychiatry unit and we tried to convince him to be admitted for a few days. He refused, so a voluntary admission was not possible. Furthermore, we had no strong documentation that he was "a threat to himself or others," so an involuntary commitment was also impossible. His obsession with his debt wouldn't go away: "So much money. So embarrassing. So ashamed. No way to repay it. Can't sleep. Can't stop pacing." He couldn't erase these thoughts from his mind, unshakable in his discontent.

About 10 months after we first saw Bernie in our clinic, his mother found him dead, on his bedroom floor. He had shot himself. We could tell that his mother was terribly sad, but she also seemed to have a sense of relief that her son's agony was over, when she reported his death to us. Her ability to cope with this tragedy was impressive, almost as if she had been preparing a long time for an unhappy ending to her son's story. The family wrote a beautiful, detailed obituary that praised his success as an engineer and even mentioned both his HD and his suicide. In the final analysis, his HD had impaired his judgement, which led to a cascade of financial mistakes, which initiated relentless anxiety and depression from which he was unable to extricate himself. We tried to help, but failed.

There are more than 1,000 suicides each year in our state and the majority are from gunshots. Bernie now joined those statistics. Our clinic team was very distressed by his death. We struggled with all the vexing questions that immediately come to mind. Could we have done more? Would a different medication have been more help? Should we have pressed him harder for a voluntary psychiatry hospitalization? Should we have been more insistent on removing his gun? There were no simple answers. We move on and try to learn from past experience. These situations are heavy burdens for everyone to bear.

Reference

1. Jamison KR. *Touched with Fire: Manic Depressive Illness and the Artistic Temperament*. Free Press, New York, 1996.

20

Staying Employed

The first symptoms of Huntington disease often begin in mid-life, precisely the time when one is just hitting his or her stride in a career path and exactly when a family most needs that earning potential. When one has HD, staying employed becomes a difficult challenge.

Sandra Smith was a 49-year-old first-grade teacher with more than two decades of experience. She was well liked by the children and highly regarded by her peers. She came to our clinic with her husband terribly concerned that her school district was threatening to fire her for incompetence. She wore wire-rimmed glasses and was a short, energetic woman with curly black hair. She produced a memo from her principal outlining her problems: Her lesson plans were disorganized. Her handwriting on the blackboard was erratic. She had left the students in the classroom unattended. Finally, she "winked and made faces" when other teachers and staff conversed with her. Little did her principal realize that he was observing the early signs of HD. Sandra was unaware of these problems and felt harassed. Her astute husband had made the connection. He pointed out that her father had died with a diagnosis of possible HD, although this was before the days of genetic testing and there was no other family history.

Sandra's examination not only showed involuntary facial movements but also the telltale twitches of her hands and body. She readily agreed to genetic testing because of its potential impact on her pending loss of job. Her genetic test revealed the mutation for HD, and our clinic genetic counselor and I agreed to meet with her school administrators to explain the turn of events.

We spent an hour in a face-to-face meeting with the superintendent, the principal and the school district's attorney. They understood that Sandra was showing the early signs of HD and, in fact, they were relieved that it wasn't drugs or alcohol or a brain tumor. Still, she could no longer teach first grade. They decided to offer her the choice of either a part-time job in another school or a medical retirement with the pension she was due.

Sandra and her husband mulled over her two choices and she decided to take the retirement. Although she was unaware of most of her disabilities, it was clear that classroom teaching had become very stressful for her and she made the right choice. She simply could no longer teach. This was a painful decision for her after nearly 30 years of identifying as a teacher. As the days passed and her anxiety level lessened, she was able to move on to a new phase of life.

■ ■ ■

William Harris was seven years younger than Sandra and a second-grade teacher in a different school district. He came to our clinic with his partner, David, seeking genetic testing. His mother and uncle had died with HD. He felt he had no symptoms, but he wanted to know if he possessed the genetic mutation so that he could make appropriate financial, career and insurance plans. He had just purchased long-term care insurance prior to seeking genetic testing. He was a tall, thin, blond gentleman with an easy smile who made perfect sense in his conversation. He had no unusual twitches and no physical or mental sign of the disease. Nevertheless, his genetic test was positive. He now knew that at some unknown point in the future he would begin to develop signs of HD.

We followed William on an annual basis. He enjoyed his teaching and had great fun interacting with the children in his class. He was a popular teacher. After about four years, he began to show subtle involuntary movements. At first, these did not interfere with his teaching and he continued as before. Slowly the movements worsened, and he eventually began to exhibit confusion and make mental mistakes. The students and parents were noticing his problems. William, like Sandra, eventually retired after a shortened but successful teaching career. He and Sandra had now entered the stage of ending their careers, living at home and accepting assistance from caring and supportive partners.

■ ■ ■

Chester Becker was a Boeing engineer—smart, focused, and a problem-solver. He did not especially want to come to the clinic, but his supervisor told him he had to seek medical advice. His work performance ratings that had gone from excellent to mediocre to poor. His supervisor thought there might be a medical problem and told him to see a doctor. Chester thought there was nothing wrong with his work performance and had a litany of excuses, including inappropriate assignments, confused schedules, and irritating fellow employees. Everyone was finding fault with him while, in his view, he was doing nothing wrong. He had, however, told the department nurse about his father dying of HD, and she advised him to see an expert.

Chester was short, bald and feisty. His speech was abrupt, almost explosive. He had clumsy hand movements and trouble with tests of balance. He was aware of no physical problems. He requested genetic testing because he understood that Boeing wanted a definitive medical diagnosis if there was one. Also, although divorced, he had a son who had just started college who would be at risk for the disease. Interestingly, the support person who came with him during the genetic testing was the company nurse. She was very helpful and supportive.

Chester's genetic test showed the HD mutation. It came as a surprise to him, and he couldn't make the connection between the test result and his problems on the job. Even so, he and the nurse took the results back to his supervisor. This led to several attempts to find him a less complicated and less stressful line of work still within the Boeing office. He tried these alternatives, but quickly failed at all of them. He simply could no longer multitask. The one advantage of these trials and failures was to convince Chester that he was no longer employable. He would not have accepted that decision when we first met. Fortunately, he had spent 30 years with the company and was eligible for a reasonable retirement package. He retired and, with other family members, began the process of selling his home and moving into a retirement community.

■ ■ ■

Jack Davenport was not as lucky. He was a truck driver. He had previously driven some big rigs, including logging trucks. These huge, long flatbed vehicles were piled high with the impressive trunks of cedar, pine or hemlock freshly cut from the massive Northwest forests. It takes strong hands, steady nerves and absolute attentiveness to successfully maneuver these rigs over twisting, mountain dirt roads. Jack did pretty well until one day he missed a curve and dumped his load. He was not injured but he lost his job. With his next truck he managed to smash a pump at a gas station, costing his company a big bill and costing Jack another job. His last assignment was driving a backhoe for a city construction crew. He backed the hoe into a tree, badly damaging both the tree and his machine. Eventually, he could no longer drive. He said it was because of his "nerves." In a way this was true; the nerves in his brain were not working properly. He floundered at home, unsuccessfully tried to kick his cigarette habit, and became completely dependent on his wife. He had no pension, but we were eventually able to convince Social Security of his obvious need for disability benefits.

Jennifer's mother had died of HD and now Jennifer was already showing signs in her early 20s. She had graduated from high school and had a job as a filing clerk in a hospital record room. When we first saw her in the clinic, she was neatly dressed in a blouse and pants, had long, brown hair and a wonderful smile. She had trouble with simple maneuvers of her fingers and difficulty moving her eyes from side to side, as well as a tendency to trip when walking. There was no doubt that her HD was symptomatic. Her filing job was the central focus of her life and the major activity of every day. Her supervisors and coworkers were absolutely magnanimous. As Jennifer's coordination and mental abilities slowly deteriorated, they provided her with all the time she needed and gave her simple tasks, clearly meant to just keep her happily occupied. This mutually agreeable arrangement went on for several years, and I think they would have always found her a place in the office. As her HD slowly progressed she could no longer walk, no longer write, and her speech was barely intelligible. Finally, she could no longer even make it to work, and her career was over. Thanks to the caring and compassion of that marvelous office staff, Jennifer has maintained a sense of dignity and self-esteem for many years. When we last saw her in a wheelchair her speech was nearly un-intelligible. There was no question she understood our conversation, and her smile and amiable personality were still evident. She died in hospice, at age 36.

■ ■ ■

Steven Robbins had spent three years in the Army. During that time he was in a motor vehicle accident, sustaining a serious head injury from which he eventually recovered. He worked his way up the administrative ladder of a local hospital to a very responsible position. His mother had died with HD and, through testing, he knew that he, too, had inherited the mutation. He came to us because of his family history of HD, and we followed him on a regular basis in our clinic. He liked to chat about the Seahawks and current events and was a practical joker. After being examined by a medical student or resident he would always enquire what they thought of his eye movements. The usual response of the student was "nothing much" or "maybe a little slow." He would then bend forward, give a little grunt, pop out his glass eye and, with a laugh, hold it in his hand for all to see. He had lost his eye following his head trauma in the Army. I don't think he demonstrated this trick for the administrator at his hospital, but he began being reprimanded for making mistakes on the job. He realized that his errors were probably the early symptoms of HD. At first, because he had no physical signs of the disease, his hospital could not see a connection between his errors of judgment and his diagnosis of HD. We were able to arrange formal neuropsychological testing by a clinical psychologist. The cognitive deficits demonstrated by this testing, combined with his family history and positive genetic test, were enough to convince his employer to give him a medical retirement rather than firing him for incompetence. This administrative result was of tremendous benefit to Steven. He wasn't fired. He wasn't labeled incompetent. He maintained his self-esteem. Also, not inconsequentially, he received medical benefits and eligibility for a pension.

21

We Just Want to Have a Child

anet's story began innocently enough. She was raised by loving parents in a large Midwestern city. She knew she was adopted, but it seemed of no consequence. She graduated from high school and college, got a good job, and married. Out of the blue, at age 25, a telephone call changed her life. The caller introduced herself as Janet's biological mother and said that she had found Janet through careful review of old adoption records that had recently been made available. She hoped they could meet. Janet and her husband thought it over and agreed to the meeting. All went well. She met both her biological mother and father. They seemed like perfectly nice people, although Janet later recalled thinking her father was "a bit odd." Her biological mother commented that she was delighted to discover Janet was "mentally normal" because there was some vague history of mental illness on her biological father's side of the family. Nothing to worry about, all families have strange characters.

Time passed and Janet's husband's job required a move to Seattle. Meanwhile, Janet was unsuccessfully trying to get pregnant. Then, two years later, another phone call spun her wheel of fortune in a new direction. It was her biological mother again. This time the news was that the mental illness on her father's side of the family had been discovered to be Huntington disease. Janet's father had just had the genetic test and it showed the HD mutation. He also was found to have symptoms and now had the diagnosis of HD. Over the phone, Janet's biological mother explained HD as best she could and relayed what she knew about genetic testing.

Janet and her husband read extensively about HD and became more and more distressed. They appeared in our clinic having made up their minds to proceed with testing. She was now 30 years old and she and her husband still very much wanted to have a child. Her biological clock was ticking. The HD diagnosis had become a new and important factor in their child planning decisions. She and her husband were very supportive of each other. In the clinic they were the kind of couple that held hands and tended to answer each other's questions.

Janet's blood was drawn, the test was done, and she and her husband returned for results. Not good news. She had inherited the gene for HD from her biological father. Clearly disappointed, she accepted the news in a calm and considerate fashion. She knew she had no symptoms or signs of HD. Uppermost in her mind was the impact of this news on their plans for having a child. She knew about prenatal diagnosis of genetic diseases and had no personal objections to abortion. She and her husband had decided that if she could get pregnant they would have prenatal diagnostic testing for HD. They obviously hoped for an unaffected child, but if the fetus had the abnormal gene for HD they would terminate the pregnancy and try again. A few months later, Janet was pregnant. She underwent prenatal genetic testing at approximately 12 weeks by chorionic villus sampling. The test was positive. The fetus had inherited the mutation for HD. They carried through their plan and terminated the pregnancy.

In a few months, Janet was pregnant again. As planned, they proceeded once again with the chorionic villus sampling drill. The chances were 50/50, just as before. The genetic coin of fate was flipped and again came up positive. This second fetus had also inherited the gene for HD. As planned, the pregnancy was terminated. Not to be denied, this couple was determined to have a child and would leave no reasonable stone unturned in obtaining that goal. They had read about the relatively new technology of preimplantation genetic diagnosis (PGD). At that time this was a new, complicated and expensive procedure which was only done at a few medical centers in this country. One of those centers was in Virginia, and Janet traveled there to begin the process.

Briefly, PGD initially involves using drugs to stimulate ovulation. Eggs are removed from the woman by a somewhat painful procedure. The eggs are fertilized in a test tube with the father's sperm. These fertilized eggs are genetically tested when they have divided to only about an eight-cell stage. Amazingly, the genetic status of the gene associated with HD can be determined in each individual fertilized egg. One or more eggs that do not have the mutation can be inserted back into the mother's uterus. With luck, since the success rate is about 25%, the egg or eggs will take hold, grow, develop and eventually produce a baby without the mutation causing HD.

At considerable time and expense, Janet completed this entire PGD experience. Unfortunately, she was not one of the lucky 25%. The egg didn't take hold and grow. She was not able to become pregnant with this procedure—yet another disappointing setback. Although one of the advantages to PGD is that the child is the product of the married mother and father, there are other possible approaches. Undaunted, Janet considered yet another option: get pregnant using a donor egg. She would not be the biological mother, but it would be her child and her husband would be the genetic, biological father. Off they went on another pregnancy adventure. An egg donor was found. The fertilized egg was placed in Janet's uterus. It did not take. There was no pregnancy. It was another failure.

The years were passing but this couple persevered. Yet another gynecologist thought one of the problems was that her uterine lining had too much scar tissue. He did a scraping procedure that was hoped to improve the uterine bed for any new fertilized egg. Meanwhile, Janet decided to forgo the issue of HD and simply try to have a child through natural means and just accept the 50% risk. It worked. The uterine scraping may have helped. She became pregnant, sailed through the pregnancy and gave birth to a little girl. There was no prenatal genetic testing and the baby might or might not have the mutation for HD. But at this point they didn't care. And yet, there was another completely unexpected spin of the genetic wheel. The little girl was not entirely normal. In fact, she had serious deficiencies of growth and development. A different kind of genetic test with chromosome studies after birth showed that she was missing an important part of one chromosome. She had a recognized syndrome called 5p-, meaning the short arm of the number five chromosome was absent. This region of the chromosome contains many important genes, and their absence results in abnormal brain development. Their new little girl may or may not have HD but definitely would have some degree of permanent brain damage. Nevertheless, they were very happy to finally have their own child.

The story doesn't end there. Janet had yet another successful pregnancy. This time she gave birth to a healthy, happy little boy. Again, there was no genetic testing. He, too, may or may not have the gene for HD, but his parents are overjoyed to have him in the family.

The years have quickly passed. Janet and her family moved back to the Midwest. Her daughter is now 11 and her son is 10. Janet herself is followed by a neurologist and has developed mild symptoms of HD. She is a stay-at-home mom and counts every day with her family as a new blessing. I have never seen a more striking example of dogged determination to have a child in spite of all the technical and genetic setbacks. Janet's coping skills are incredible. She sees her story as one of determined persistence and eventual success. Who can disagree? Janet's struggle to have a child began with the discovery that her biological father had HD. In the next chapter we will meet Vicki, whose similar discovery had very different consequences.

22

The Judge Said, "Are You Sure You Want to Do This?"

The Skagit Valley, north of Seattle, is a tranquil landscape of rolling green hills alternating with flat farmland enriched by centuries of flooding by the Skagit River meandering through the valley. To the west is the shoreline of Puget Sound, which is popular with boaters and provides an entrance to the enchanting San Juan Islands. To the east are the snow-caped Cascade Mountains. In the valley between these two impressive landmarks one can find dairy farms and thousands of acres of daffodil and tulip fields. In April and May there is a carpet of yellow, purple, red and pink flowers spreading to the distant horizon with the white cone of the dormant volcano Mt. Baker guarding the region as a distant sentinel to the north. Because of the area's natural popularity with tourists, William and Evelyn VanDuser were able to operate a successful bed and breakfast in one of the small towns that dot the valley. They lived there with their daughter Vicki, who attended the local high school and cheerfully helped with duties around the B&B. Vicki was an average student, played trumpet in the band, and was popular with the other kids. She was full of energy and had a penchant for getting into trouble, although never anything serious. William and Evelyn were pleased that she graduated on time, but were uncertain where she was headed next. Vicki was certain that she wanted to get out of the isolated village and quickly moved to Seattle where she got a job clerking in a clothing store. On a whim, she bought a motorcycle and soon fell in with a crowd doing drugs. Her experiment with drugs only lasted a few months. She entered an outpatient rehab program and was soon "clean" and back on track. However, by age 24 she lost concentration, started making too many mistakes on the job, and was fired. Her friends told her that she was talking "funny," had developed an irritating facial twitch, and should go see a doctor. Her doctor agreed that something was wrong and referred her to a neurologist.

Vicki was nervous about the neurology appointment and asked her parents to go with her. The neurologist was cordial, organized, and systematically reviewed her story. When the doctor asked about family history Vicki shrugged her shoulders and matter-of-factly said she was adopted and had no family history. Neither Vicki nor the doctor realized that this simple question stunned Vicki's parents, who were suddenly jolted back in time.

Going back 24 years, William and Evelyn had lived in Seattle, where William was a mechanical engineer helping to build airplanes for the Boeing company and Evelyn was an elementary school teacher. They were happily married but frustrated by not being able to have children. One day, their friends the Smiths brought home a month-old baby girl they planned to raise as a foster child. They named her Victoria and called her Vicki. For William and Evelyn it was love at first sight. Vicki was exactly the child they had been hoping for. They discussed their instant attraction to the baby with the Smiths, who said they had no long-term plans for Vicki and encouraged William and Evelyn to adopt her. They began having excited discussions with the Catholic adoption agency in charge of the child. During one of their meetings an agency employee told them the records showed that Vicki's mother was a 17-year-old unmarried woman who had a family history of Huntington's chorea. William and Evelyn knew nothing about the disease, were obviously curious and asked about it. The woman told them she also knew very little but understood it was a genetic condition and that Vicki's mother did not seem to have it. She also understood that Vicki might not inherit it and, in any event, there was no way to tell. This limited, second-hand information was good enough for William and Evelyn. In their enthusiasm to move forward with the adoption they had no interest in learning more about some rare, obscure genetic disease. They also knew the baby had passed her pediatric medical exam with flying colors. They felt safe.

The adoption process was frustratingly slow. Finally, when Vicki was six months old, William and Evelyn had an appointment with a judge to sign the final adoption papers. They were nervous and excited. The judge was an elderly, stoic gentleman who was all business and didn't engage in small talk. As he sat behind his massive desk and rustled through the adoption papers he suddenly paused, looked up, and said, "This says the baby has a family history of Huntington's chorea? Did you know that?" Evelyn replied that yes, the adoption agency had mentioned something about HD. The judge remarked that he had seen several persons with the disease. He noted that it was a brain illness and could be very serious. He also knew that it was hereditary. William said they knew that, but they were told that Vicki's mother didn't seem to have it. Further, he mentioned that Vicki's physical exam was normal and that she might well not have inherited the disease. The judge looked directly at them and said, "Are you sure you want to do this?" William and Evelyn both quickly agreed that yes, they loved Vicki and dearly wanted to adopt her as their daughter. The papers were signed and off they went.

Now, 24 years later in the neurologist's office, William and Evelyn revealed they had been told Vicki's biological mother had a family history of Huntington's chorea. This was news to Vicki, who had no idea what that meant. The neurologist, of course, knew exactly what it meant. She took time to give the family a quick overview of HD and concluded that it might well explain Vicki's present social and cognitive problems. The neurologist ordered an MRI brain scan and a genetic blood test. The brain scan was normal, but the genetic test revealed the mutation associated with HD. The surprise of the HD diagnosis was unsettling. Vicki seemed to realize she was going to have trouble finding employment and making it on her own. She returned to the B&B in the Skagit River Valley to live with her parents, and they began educating themselves about HD.

Over the next few years Vicki's movements slowly worsened. The medications tried by the doctor were not much help. She wanted to be proactive and so signed up for a research project investigating HD at the National Institutes of Health (NIH). Vicki flew back to Bethesda, Maryland, for the study, all expenses paid. She was there for four days and underwent an exhausting series of blood tests, physical exams, psychological tests, brain scans and a spinal tap. In the waiting room of the NIH clinic Vicki struck up a conversation with a young man taking part in a completely separate research study of brain tumors. They discovered Bethesda was pretty boring so they went to dinner and spent the evenings together. When their studies ended they parted ways, never to see each other again.

A few weeks after returning home, Vicki discovered she was pregnant. She was not particularly interested in having a baby, but she was also strictly against termination of the pregnancy. Nine months later she gave birth to a healthy eight-pound boy and named him Phillip. Soon after the delivery Vicki's disease began producing disabling psychiatric symptoms. She had long periods of apathy alternating with episodes of agitated mania. She showed little interest in caring for her baby. William and Evelyn realized that raising Phillip was going to be their job. They were going to be parents of a small child once again.

Vicki's behavior worsened. She thought she was being attacked by insects. She became paranoid and became suspicious that everyone was plotting against her. One day, she packed a small suitcase and vanished. William and Evelyn notified the police but were unable to find her. Much later they learned that she had moved into a homeless tent camp in Seattle. She never returned home and they lost all contact with her.

Meanwhile, William and Evelyn turned their attention to raising little Phillip. They decided to pool their savings, sell their B&B, move to a larger city, and devote themselves to their grandson. He was an exuberant boy and they were delighted to watch him grow and develop. They were, however, hyper-alert to signs of HD. By the time he was 11 years old he had been playing on a baseball team for three years. His grandparents began to notice that he was losing skills rather than gaining new ones. They became very concerned and took him to a doctor and a genetics counselor. They related Vicki's story and said they wanted Phillip tested for HD. The medical team was reluctant to do genetic testing because his neurological exam was normal and they thought it would be better to wait and see if there were any further changes. Their general protocol was not to test children at risk for HD unless they had more telltale signs of the disease, such as chorea. They wanted to avoid unnecessarily labeling a child as having HD because of possible negative emotional and social consequences. The child might be treated as "different" or "abnormal."

Over the next two years Phillip not only lost the ability to play baseball but also had a behavioral change. He became argumentative, short-tempered and began to fight with his classmates and even his grandparents. William and Evelyn took him to a child psychologist, who then sent him back to the genetics clinic. This time it was agreed to proceed with testing. Sadly, his test result returned positive. The size of the DNA expansion in his HD gene was more than 80 repeats. He had inherited HD from his mother, just as she had from her mother. In fact, Phillip had juvenile HD.

The disease slowly took its toll on Phillip, but his symptoms were mostly physical. Strangely, he had another personality change, this time for the better. He became mellow, relaxed, and quite affable. Phillip's classmates and teachers rallied to his cause and surrounded him with a network of marvelous support, just as happened to Bobbi with juvenile HD, in Chapter 16. When he made it to high school they began to call him "Prince Phillip." He became a school celebrity. Everyone knew and liked Prince Phillip. By then he was in a wheelchair and needed extra time to pass his special classes, but pass them he did. At age 20, in cap and flowing green gown, he received his diploma from the principal while all his classmates stood and cheered. His grandfather William had died of cancer two years before, but Evelyn was immensely proud of her grandson.

Juvenile HD is notorious for being more rapidly progressive than the adult variety. Phillip's experience was no exception. Following his high school graduation he soon entered an adult care home requiring round-the-clock services. His body became stiff and rigid, his speech was difficult to understand, and he began having trouble swallowing. He entered hospice care and died at age 22.

I interviewed Evelyn about 50 years after she and William had adopted Vicki. She still vividly recalled the judge asking them, "Are you sure you want to do this?" Little did they know what the future held in store for them. Of course, that's true of every adoption, indeed of every child, adopted or not. Evelyn was glad they had done what they had done. Yes, they were sure.

23

The Thanksgiving Visitor

Family holidays are supposed to be full of good feelings and joyful celebration, but they can also be charged with stress and tension. Many families recognize the iconic cartoonish uncle who sits at the holiday table and bloviates his outlandish and embarrassing ideas. The Smith family had no loutish uncle to contend with. At their Thanksgiving feast they had to deal with Huntington disease.

The November weather was crisp and clear when Melissa arrived on time for the family gathering. Her mother, Margaret, had invited her home for Thanksgiving, but was actually surprised when she appeared. Melissa had HD and was living in a homeless shelter. She had been adopted as an infant and the family did not learn of her biological mother's diagnosis of HD until Melissa was graduating from high school. Her life as a young adult had been chaotic. In retrospect, the family realized that her frequent judgmental and behavioral lapses were early signs of HD. She had a child, Billy, and quickly separated from the boy's unreliable father. She was unable to care for an infant, turned Billy over to her parents, and became a homeless wanderer. She would disappear for long stretches. Recently, Margaret discovered that Melissa was living in a shelter not far from home. She was paying for Melissa's cell phone so, on a sudden whim, she called and invited her for Thanksgiving. Now she had arrived and the tension in the house was palpable.

Melissa had little to say and essentially interacted with no one. Little Billy, now five years old, seemed excited to see her. He tried to entice her to come see his newly decorated bedroom. She refused. He was greatly disappointed, cried for a moment but, being a very sociable kid, wandered off to play with other relatives. Melissa hugged her purse tightly to her side the entire afternoon. Her mother suspected she was worried that it might be stolen. Paranoid ideas would not be new for Melissa. At mealtime she refused to sit at the table and refused to eat. This was not too surprising to Margaret because Melissa had previously accused the family of trying to poison her. When other family members were watching football on TV, Melissa silently stood off to the side staring blankly across the room with that familiar thousand-mile stare. The occasional twitches of her body were not especially noticeable unless you closely watched her. When someone tried to engage her in conversation she said, "Leave me alone." When her sister touched her arm she quickly withdrew and exclaimed, "Don't you touch me."

After a few hours of negligible social interactions, Melissa declared it was time to leave. Margaret offered to drive her to the shelter with Billy and went to the closet to retrieve their coats. When she returned she found Melissa already out the door walking toward a car parked at the curb. Margaret realized that Melissa wanted nothing to do with a family drive and had called an Uber. In a melancholy mood, Margaret stood quietly at the living room window watching the car slowly pull away and disappear around the corner. She tried to make sense of the afternoon's events, her thoughts tumbling through her mind: "What just happened? That's not the girl I used to know. That is a different person. The old Melissa is gone. I hope she will be safe. I wonder that will happen if she returns for Christmas? I wonder what's in store for Billy? What unbelievable ways this Huntington's disease has changed our family."

24

Family Opposites

Rachael Morgan was born in Omaha, Nebraska, in 1938. Her childhood was unremarkable. There were family picnics in the hot Nebraska summers and snow sledding with her neighborhood friends in the winter. Family finances were stretched thin in the late years of the Depression, but in the post–World War II era they could afford a powder-blue '49 Pontiac and a family trip to Chicago. Rachael was outgoing and friendly and did well in school. During high school she had frequent arguments with her mother, who seemed to quickly lose her temper. Their arguments seemed to be the usual adolescent rebellion versus parental angst. Rachael never knew her maternal grandfather; he died in the State Mental Hospital when she was in middle school. If he had a neurological diagnosis, she didn't know it.

After graduating from high school, Rachael went to the University of Iowa, where she joined a sorority and received excellent grades. In fact, she was listed in the 1958 edition of "Who's Who in American Colleges." She graduated with a degree in home economics and considered becoming a high school teacher. Instead, at 23, she married a charming young man, Peter, who worked as a bank teller, and a year later they had a son. The marriage did not go well. Looking back on things, the family now realizes that Rachael had a slow but clear personality change in her 20s. Outside the home she continued to be pleasant with friends and neighbors, but was most unpleasant with her family. Seemingly out of nowhere, her temper descended into her life and rarely retreated. Little things irritated her and she lost her temper nearly every day. She argued with her husband and fought with her son. Mealtimes were a disaster and she had a temper tantrum nearly every night. Her degree in home economics was not helping. The marriage crumbled and ended in divorce after six years. Taking her son with her, she returned to Omaha to live with her parents.

Unfortunately, returning home did not work. The adolescent scraps she had experienced with her mother started up where they had left off and only worsened. She and her mother seemed to have the same irritable disagreeable personality. They fought about clothes, they fought about food, they fought over money, and they fought over childcare. Rachael's father was at a loss and just tried to stay out of the way. Her retreat to the expected welcoming childhood home soon became intolerable.

Rachael had kept in touch with Peter and pleaded to return to him. Against his better judgement, but wanting to see his son again and remembering the Rachael of a decade ago, he accepted her back. In fact, they remarried. To no one's surprise it didn't work. The fighting and anger and temper tantrums all returned. Rachael's brain was disconnecting. Peter didn't understand what was happening, but he realized he had made a mistake and within a year they again divorced.

Given her unhappy home life it was intriguing how well Rachael was able to control her behavior in the community. To this degree, the ebb and flow of her emotions was predictable. She continued to have friends and joined the PTA. When she was out shopping, the clerks and storekeepers would have no idea of her smoldering anxiety and unhappiness. She was able to maintain that outer composure so well that she met another man, Norman, and they soon married. She and Norman had her second son, and his job required a move to Texas. Meanwhile, back in Omaha, Rachael's mother had a progressive, serious physical and mental deterioration that put her in a nursing home, where she died at age 62. Her doctors suspected that she and her father, Rachael's grandfather, had Huntington disease, but this news did not make its way to Rachael.

In Texas, Norman was shocked when he discovered the "real" Rachael he hadn't known. Her temper tantrums at home only worsened. She smashed dishes on the floor and threw furniture against the wall. She hit Norman and both children, luckily without serious injury. She began to sleep during much of the day and have prolonged screaming fits at night. Sometimes she would be quiet and uncommunicative and at other times erupt with rapid nonsensical chattering and singing. More than once she ran screaming into the neighborhood at night and the police were called to shepherd her home. She became sloppy and uncaring about her personal appearance. Her hair was uncombed, her dress untidy, and her clothes frequently unwashed. At other times she would wander naked around the house. She also became a pack rat. Nothing was thrown away. The house began to fill up with junk of all sorts: pieces of clothing, old unused toys, unwashed dishes and silverware, unread paperback books, empty grocery bags, newspapers and magazines. The house, attic and garage all overflowed with trash. She spread newspapers around the floor in some strange attempt at cleanliness. Norman and the boys never let anyone visit their home. Norman carefully brought all of this behavior to the attention of her family doctor, who prescribed tranquilizers. Rachael refused to take them. Her two sons kept out of the house as much as possible, staying in school, going to community activities, joining Boy Scouts, or playing at friends' houses. When Rachael was in her early 40s, Norman's business required another move, this time to Seattle. Norman recalls that it was around this time that he first noted physical signs of deterioration in Rachael. Her coordination was off. She frequently stumbled and sometimes dropped dishes. Her speech became slurred and garbled. A few years later, when she attended her oldest son's wedding, the other guests whispered and raised their eyebrows over her boisterous, unpredictable behavior. They assumed she had spent too much time at the punch bowl.

In her late 40s, Norman was able to have Rachael seen by a psychiatrist who put her behavior, clumsiness and family history together and made the diagnosis of Huntington disease. Norman and the sons were shocked by the diagnosis. Yet, when they learned about the disease, they realized that it all made sense. Rachael continued to refuse medication and her involuntary movements became more flagrant. One day, she fell on the stairs, hit her head, lost consciousness, and was quickly hospitalized. Neurosurgeons removed a large blood clot from underneath her skull (subdural hematoma) and she regained consciousness. She was sent to a nursing home for rehabilitation, where she slowly began to walk again. After a few weeks she slipped, fell, slammed her head on the floor and again lost consciousness. Back at the hospital studies showed the blood clots were now on both sides of the brain, larger than ever. The doctors were reluctant to reoperate and she died the next day, at age 55.

■ ■ ■

Rachael's second son was Benjamin. When he was an infant, Norman feared for Ben's well-being. Rachael would sometimes cradle Ben in her left arm as she threw objects at Norman with her right hand. Norman was afraid she might throw Ben. She never did. She never physically injured Ben. The psychological injury would be harder to measure. As he grew older, Ben became adept at avoiding his mother. He enjoyed school, stayed out of trouble and was a good student. In high school his grades were 4.0 and he was a proud member of the National Honor Society. Easily accepted into the University of Washington, he moved to an apartment near campus. Finally he was on his own, away from the frightful environment of his mother.

College work was harder than Ben had anticipated. He got a few decent grades, but he lost interest in his studies. He couldn't concentrate. His grades suffered. He told his father he wanted to be a rock star. He quit college and took a job as a waiter in a restaurant. He tried to play the guitar but slowly discovered he had no musical talent. Waiting on tables lasted about a year. He was fired for being undependable and having too many absences. Ben returned to college where he passed a few courses and failed a few. Again he dropped out of school and tried low entry-level jobs: Burger King, Walmart, and Dairy Queen. None of these lasted more than a few months. He could not stick to a schedule and was repeatedly fired for missing too much work. Once again he returned to college and slowly accumulated course credits. He switched from a business major to English. He struggled for two years trying to pass the foreign language requirement. He picked Latin because it was a dead language that he would not have to speak. Finally, after eight stop-and-start years, he was a college graduate.

What did the future hold for an unmotivated English major who knew a few words of Latin? He got a job as cashier at Fred Meyer. Mostly he wanted to listen to music all night and sleep in the next morning. His cashier job lasted a year and then he was fired again. Meanwhile, Ben's father had remarried. When Ben's new stepmother met him she quickly recognized something was wrong. He was not behaving like a National Honor Society graduate. He was incredibly apathetic, without motivation or ambition. Norman and his new wife decided it was time to find out if HD was playing a role in Ben's deteriorating life. Ben shrugged his shoulders and passively agreed to be evaluated.

Ben's first clinic visit was uneventful. The doctors and counselors saw an apathetic, introverted young man who was attentive but spoke in monosyllables and seemed disinterested. He was tall and heavyset with smooth skin and a crew cut. He acted more like a shy 14-year-old teenager than a 30-year-old man. It was also noted that he had no involuntary movements. He clearly understood his 50% risk for HD. His father remembered that a blood sample had been collected and banked from Ben's mother Rachael, just before her death. The sample had been sent to another hospital, but it was retrieved and so two samples were sent to the lab. Both test results returned positive. Rachael had 44 CAG repeats in the *HTT* gene and Ben had 48. When he heard the result, Ben's only question was whether this meant he was going to start behaving like his mother. The guarded answer was "not necessarily." Surprisingly, that answer turned out to be entirely accurate.

Ben's parents set him up in an apartment and tried to carefully monitor his activities. He had clearly shown that he was unemployable and eventually qualified for Social Security Disability payments. He spent most of his time by himself, although he would occasionally wander to the local library or bookstore. There he would sit for hours, staring at a book or magazine, rarely turning the pages. He mostly continued his cycle of sleeping during the day and listening to music or watching TV all night. For a while he became interested in building and painting model ships and airplanes. One day he proudly showed the clinic staff a destroyer and jet fighter that he had spent weeks gluing and painting, once again seeming like that 14-year-old boy. His smile radiated a child's sense of accomplishment in proudly showing off his models. As the years went by, he began to develop chorea and his coordination suffered. He could no longer construct the models. His parents lived about 15 miles away and visited him several times a week. He had a microwave and his father stocked his small refrigerator with TV dinners. His father also took him on drives and sometimes they went to a movie.

Ben avoided interacting with other people. He never got angry, never argued, and never lost his temper. He fell into the role of a quiet loner. Once when visiting his parents he wandered out into the night and disappeared. They frantically looked for him, but he couldn't be found. They reported his disappearance to the police, who also couldn't find him. The next day, Norman's phone rang and he feared the worst. Maybe Ben's body had been found along a back road. Instead, the call was from Ben. He had walked the 15 miles in the dark back to his apartment, simply because he decided it was time to go home. It's a mystery how he found his way home that night, but there he was, back in his comfort zone, watching TV. Now in his early 40s, Ben remains a shy but reasonably happy and content man living a secluded and sheltered life under the watchful eyes of his aging parents.

■ ■ ■

When I am asked to describe a "typical" patient with HD I often think of Rachael and Ben. Neither of them is exactly typical of HD, nor is anyone else. In fact, one theme of this book is the never-ending variety of behavior shown by people with this disease. Yet, taken together, Rachael and Ben show two common sides of the HD coin. On the one hand, there is Rachael's personality change, irritability, dramatic mood swings, antisocial behavior, and compulsive hoarding, finally combined with clumsiness and eventually leading to head trauma and death. On the other hand, there is Ben's apathy, loss of motivation, inability to hold a job, and withdrawal into lonely isolation. Were it not for his parents, Ben would certainly be homeless. It remains fascinating and unexplained how two people with the same disease, so close to each other in the same family, could exhibit such completely different personalities. Together, they cover a lot of the behaviors seen within the HD spectrum.

And then there was Rachael's husband, Norman. For more than 40 years he cared first for his wife and then a son with HD. Consistently. Patiently. Quietly. Without complaint. He was yet another caregiver unexpectedly caught in the web of HD. As Linda Loman said, "Attention must be paid."

25

A Second Wedding

Michael was a busy and successful business man overseeing a large portfolio of real estate contracts. In his 40s he had developed some nervous twitches that seemed of no consequence and were written off as just an expected part of his high-stress and anxiety-producing job. By age 51, his family doctor thought the movements were too odd to be ignored and sent him on to a neurologist. The neurologist thought the twitches might be chorea and, even though he had no family history of chorea, the genetic blood test for HD was ordered. Michael and his wife Marie were stunned when the result came back positive. They went through several months of the not unexpected stages of denial, anger, and eventually grudging acceptance. Michael had the good fortune of having been in the Air Force and was eligible for additional medical services at the VA Hospital. These VA resources proved of considerable benefit in terms of helping to pay for medications and providing periods of respite care for Michael several years down the road.

But, when I first met this couple in the clinic, I was fearful that the new devastating diagnosis of HD might ruin their marriage, as described with some of the other couples in the previous chapters. I needn't have worried. Over the subsequent months and years HD actually seemed to strengthen their relationship. In fact, they decided to have a formal "convalidation" of their marriage. They went all out and had a full ceremony at St. John the Evangelist Catholic Church. The pews were full of 200 smiling friends and relatives. There were neckties and corsages as well as a few work shirts and jeans. All were welcome. Bouquets of white lilies and pink dahlias were on either side of the altar. The couple's four-year-old son slowly walked down the aisle as the somewhat dazed but happy ring bearer. A great joy was felt throughout the church. Marie, lovely in her bridal gown, and Michael, in his tux, said their vows and exchanged kisses. I was worried that this moment would be a problem for Michael because he tended to have an idiosyncratic kind of chorea that caused irregularity of his diaphragm and frequent grunts and sudden pauses while speaking. I was delighted to see him triumph over this problem with a smiling face and a clear voice. Several years later I was reminded of Michael's marriage vows when watching the movie *The King's Speech*, dramatizing George VI's triumph over his severe stuttering when giving his radio address to the English people at the onset of World War II. Michael was every bit as good as King George. Well done, Michael.

Marie spent the next decade struggling with Michael's slow but unremitting deterioration. Finally, after many false starts in poorly run adult family homes, they found a nursing facility in Seattle that gave excellent care. In a talk to the staff, this is how Marie described their journey, in her own words. With her permission, I have included her message verbatim because of its heartfelt personal description of a life with HD.

If someone had told me 21 years ago when I married my husband, Michael, that I would be here tonight talking about his nursing home, there's a good chance I would have left him at the altar. I'm glad I didn't know what was in store for us, because I would have missed an incredible journey rich with unexpected blessings. One of those blessing is Bailey-Boushay House.

Thirteen years ago, we learned that Michael had something called Huntington's disease. We'd never heard of it. His doctor gave him the news, handed him a copy of a page from *The Big Book of Bad Diseases* and sent him on his way with our four-year-old son in tow. We read and re-read that paragraph describing HD—what's burned in my memory are seven words: devastating, degenerative, neurological—no cure/no treatment.

Over the years we've learned a lot about HD—up close and personal as Michael would say. I've witnessed the devastating effects of this disease take their toll not only on my husband, but our entire family. Once an avid cyclist, now just being pushed around the block in his wheelchair exhausted him. Witty & articulate, social & outgoing, a world traveler—Michael's world now consisted of watching TV in the family room. He could no longer read or chat on the phone with his few remaining friends. It's a lonely, isolating disease.

I'd been warned early on that eventually, every person afflicted with HD would require full-time care. It wasn't a matter of if Michael would be institutionalized, but when. If that wasn't bad enough, to top it off, very few nursing facilities would even take HD patients. I became his full-time caregiver. I wasn't his wife anymore—I was his nurse. He was no longer my husband, but a patient with a very challenging and complicated disease. I was also working full time and running a household and raising our two boys. I was emotionally and physically exhausted—I didn't like who I was when I was around Michael—and I was with him 24 hours a day. I wanted better for all of us.

So, one year ago yesterday, Michael moved out of the home and away from the family we had begun 20 years earlier. I'll give you only the highlights of the first 3½ months—it would take way too long to tell you everything that happened in that short span. His first two months were spent in an adult family home. Following a temper tantrum that stay culminated with him being transported to Harborview Hospital, locked in handcuffs, where he stayed for *a day before being sent to the VA hospital for a two-week stay. He was then transferred to an understaffed nursing home in the "transitional room" (euphemism for holding cell) while we waited for a room to come available at Bailey-Boushay House, a nursing home for patients with complex problems.*

I knew about Bailey through a couple we had met at our first HD support group back in 1997—Tom and Virginia. I remember that day like it was yesterday. Seeing Tom, Michael got a glimpse of his future—random, spastic movements, unintelligible speech, grimacing facial expressions. It was too much—he put his head on the table and cried. HD now had a face—it was real. As I watched Virginia and Tom interact, I was struck by the love they shared, how patient, kind and compassionate she was. I knew that if we could hold onto the love, we'd make it. To be honest—after 13 years, I'd lost that loving feeling.

About two years ago Tom moved to Bailey-Boushay. I had kept in touch with Virginia and had followed their odyssey to Bailey—they found it after moving from place to place, much like Michael. They were happy at Bailey, Tom loved it there. In talking about the staff at Bailey, Virginia said, "They get it." That's all I needed to hear. HD is a complicated disease. If they "got it" they were in the minority. It must be a special place.

Michael has lived at the Bailey-Boushay for 8½ months. From the moment we entered the lobby, we knew this was a special place. This was the Hilton of care facilities. Not only is it a lovely facility, the staff is happy, smiling and accommodating, from the receptionist to the executive director. They accepted Michael with no hesitation.

The nightmare of the past three months had left Michael fearful and combative. He reminded me of a caged animal, if you were in striking distance, it was likely you'd get hit. It broke my heart. At home, I would dread the phone call, one I had received many times from those other places, telling me to get down there and calm my husband down, or they'd call 911. I never got that call. But I was nervous when I attended the first care conference arranged by Michael's care manager, Sally. She said that the staff psychiatrist as well as the executive director would be there. I figured they were going to warn me in person rather than over the phone. I was so afraid we'd be asked to leave this wonderful place we'd found. I sat down, and the first thing the director said was (I'm paraphrasing), "First of all, I want you to know that you're not in trouble. We want Michael to stay here and we will do whatever it takes to make it work. This is his home for as long as he wants to stay here." I think I cried—they were tears of relief. Finally, I could breathe. For the first time in years, I felt the burden lift—I wasn't alone. I was surrounded by people who genuinely cared about Michael, who wanted to know Michael the person—not Michael the disease. For over an hour we strategized. The psychiatrist addressed the myriad of medications Michael was taking and suggested some new therapies. Sally, wonderful Sally, took notes as I told them about my husband. They actively listened. I left feeling hopeful—there was light at the end of the tunnel. Now to be perfectly honest, I was a little skeptical. It's one thing to strategize – but would they implement those strategies? And would they work?

The very next day when I came to visit Michael, he seemed different, he was smiling and peaceful. I didn't see fear in his eyes. He pointed to the wall in front of him. The first sign to catch my eye read "I'm Michael and I have Huntington's Disease. Please be patient with me." Everything we had talked about in that meeting had materialized. Instructions to staff about Michael's needs; his daily routine listed on a whiteboard. (Routine and order is very important for someone with HD.) I followed Michael's gaze to a poster Sally had made for him. You see, she took time to talk to Michael, to find what was really important to him, to get to know him. Here's what is written on that poster: "I'm proud to be the father of two amazing sons. I'm proud to have been a supportive husband for 20 years. I'm proud to be able to feed myself. I'm proud to be Catholic and to pray. Finally, I'm proud to be sober for 26 years." No longer did he have to struggle to be understood—if you wanted to know Michael, all you had to do was look at the wall. That was the turning point. His fear and anxiety were lifted. Now if you're within striking distance of Michael, all you'll get is a hug, a smile and "I love you!"

I'm Michael's wife again and I'm feeling the love. We've experienced some normal moments at Bailey. Curling up together and *watching It's a Wonderful Life on Christmas day with our boys. Or this summer visiting with Tom and Virginia on the deck at Bailey. For a little while we weren't caregivers and patients. We were an ordinary couple chatting in the sunshine on a beautiful Seattle Saturday afternoon.*

We're fortunate to have been able to spend time with Tom—his room was just a couple doors down from Michael's. They have a lot in common far beyond HD. Incredible strength, faith and perseverance in the face of seemingly insurmountable odds. Tom's cool—Michael would say. Sadly, Tom passed away a few weeks ago. I was touched by the compassion and love of the staff, allowing Tom to leave this earth with grace and dignity. We'll miss him. I'll be forever grateful for the day they came into our lives. Yet another blessing in disguise.

I don't know what the future holds, but I know that as long as Michael is at Bailey, we're going to be okay.

Michael eventually lost his ability to speak clearly and two years later died of pneumonia. He remained content and happy up to the end, giving a smile and a hug to all his visitors.

The two marriages, of George and Kay (in Chapter 18) and now Michael and Marie, show both couples dealing with HD in flexible and accommodating ways. They exemplify the strength of love and companionship facing unexpected and potentially devastating challenges with impressive composure and courage.

To have and to hold from this day forward
For better, for worse
For richer, for poorer
In sickness and in health
Til death do us part.

PART IV

Embarrassment, Injury, Neglect and Delusions

Persons with Huntington disease are often unaware of their involuntary movements. When brought to their attention, these movements can be embarrassing or lead to social ostracism. Accusations of drug abuse or intoxication are common. The muscle incoordination can also result in serious bodily harm. Broken bones, automobile crashes, head trauma, and house fires can all result from this disease.

Furthermore, the obvious chorea and lack of sound judgment may make the individual with HD highly vulnerable to abuse and neglect. Persons with HD can be found in the homeless population on our city streets. Without a protective care group, persons with HD can be taken advantage of, with serious consequences.

The mental aberrations sometimes associated with the disease can lead to disturbing delusions, sometimes as severe as fear of diabolical possession. The sum of the accumulating symptoms can lead to a downward physical and emotional spiral that requires a strong network of support to prevent unnecessary harm. The following vignettes will illustrate many of these dangers.

26

"Excuse Me, Madam" and "I Am Not Drunk"

It can be startling to suddenly realize that other people see you as peculiar. A case in point is Marilyn, who had always assumed she was healthy. One Saturday afternoon, she was doing some last-minute shopping in her local grocery store. Out of nowhere a spectacled white-haired gentleman approached her and said, "Excuse me, madam, but I am a retired doctor and notice that you have chorea. Did you know you have chorea?"

Taken aback, Marilyn stammered, "I don't know what you mean."

The elderly man continued: "I mean you have involuntary movements called chorea and you need to see a neurologist. I will give you a note to take to your family doctor that says that you need to see a neurologist. It is important."

The man proceeded to take a small black notebook from one pocket and a silver pen from another. He leaned against a cabinet and, as if dashing off a prescription, wrote the following note: "This woman has chorea and it is my opinion she needs to see a neurologist. EB Jones, MD."

He carefully tore out the page, folded it and handed it to Marilyn. He said, "Be sure and give this to your doctor. It is very important." Touching her on the arm and giving a slight bow he disappeared around the next aisle.

Marilyn was surprised and confused. Dr. Jones was an apparition speaking a different language. She had no idea what he was talking about. She wondered what he saw about her that was different. Nevertheless, he seemed serious and sincere, so she actually did what he requested. Her family doctor agreed she had some involuntary movements, but did not think she could possibly have Huntington chorea. He had never seen a case, but knew the disease was hereditary and Marilyn could think of no family member with neurological or mental problems. However, the consulting neurologist who saw her next became more suspicious of HD when he realized that Marilyn knew nothing about her father or his side of the family because he had left her mother when Marilyn was two years old. Sure enough, the genetic test revealed the mutation associated with HD. A chance occurrence in a grocery store led to a life-changing event for Marilyn. It could have been different. Instead of her being advised by an observant retired doctor, the store manager could have had asked her to leave because she appeared intoxicated. This is what happened to Mr. Barkley.

■ ■ ■

The vast majority of persons with HD are not alcoholic. However, they do have poor coordination and sudden movements they cannot control, making them appear intoxicated to the casual observer. This can cause all sorts of public embarrassment and even confrontations.

Mr. Barkley was a successful attorney who was married and had a six-year-old daughter, Sarah. He developed his first symptoms of HD in his 40s. His left shoulder would twitch, then his right hand, and he was constantly winking and blinking. Using stairs was a problem. He would often trip and stumble. After four years of progressively worsening symptoms HD had forced him into semi-retirement, although he was spending two days a week at the office.

On one of his days off, Mr. Barkley took Sarah to the local shopping center where she found her favorite playground. Her father blended in with the shopping mall crowd, although his hair was uncombed and one shoe was untied. He carefully watched her, sometimes standing close by and other times sitting on a bench. The shoppers shuffled up and down the wide aisles, seemingly oblivious to the playground. After about 30 minutes, a shopping center police officer approached and confronted him, asked him for his ID and questioned what he was doing. Someone had pointed him out as being a suspicious character hanging around the children's playground. Being a very articulate man, Mr. Barkley explained himself and that he was the father of the little girl. He also mentioned that he had a disease that affected his coordination. The policeman remained suspicious and probably suspected he was intoxicated. The officer insisted they telephone his wife, who was able to confirm his story. Of course, little Sarah was frightened and confused about the whole episode and her father was aghast and terribly embarrassed.

■ ■ ■

Being accused of public intoxication is a recurring theme in the life of persons with HD and worth exploring with a few more examples.

One man with HD was pulled over to the side while driving because his brake lights were not working. The officer thought his speech was slurred, had him step out of the car, and asked him to walk a straight line. He failed this test and the policeman concluded he was driving while intoxicated. Although his breathalyzer test was negative, this did not change the officer's assumption. The man was arrested and it took several phone calls back and forth with our office before he was finally released. He still had to appear later in court with a letter for the judge explaining the mistaken assumption.

I have also seen persons with HD stopped for driving erratically and accused of being drunk. They were not drunk, but they were driving erratically. The distinction is important, but does not absolve the person of poor driving. In fact, as with many other neurological disorders, the time often arises when the person with HD should no longer be driving. I once had a patient with HD who had had several fender benders and whose chorea and incoordination were quite obvious. I filled out the appropriate Department of Motor Vehicles form recommending that this individual no longer be allowed to drive, for both her safety and the safety of the public. The logical response of the Department was to give her a formal driving test, which she proudly passed; she remained behind the wheel for another two years. Sometimes one's best intentions go for naught. I couldn't imagine her parallel parking, but apparently she did.

■ ■ ■

One man with chorea could not make it past a Metro bus driver. His jerks and twitches caused him to fumble badly with his change and he could not insert the coins into the money box. The driver thought he was intoxicated and gave him an order: "Get off my bus!" There was no way he would win that argument, especially with a dozen riders staring at him and getting increasingly angry that an alcoholic was delaying their morning commute. Surprised and dejected, he reluctantly returned to the street corner hoping to regain his composure and try again with another bus.

■ ■ ■

One evening, Monica Brewer was standing on the sidewalk waiting to enter a jazz club. She was animatedly chatting with her neighbors in line. A passing patrolman noticed her uncoordinated movements and informed her that she was under arrest for public intoxication. She began to argue and explain that it was a neurological problem, not alcohol. Monica was a feisty character and during the ensuing argument her involuntary movements caused her to physically bump the officer more than once. He added attempted assault to the charges and she was taken to jail, where she spent several restless nights. She was given a trial date and faced the possibility of more weeks or even months in jail. Fortunately, she found a reasonable defense attorney who took the time to contact us and got a better understanding of Monica's disease. Our clinic social worker and I explained HD and chorea to the attorney and provided a detailed letter of explanation. The lawyer agreed to use involuntary movements as the defense, but even with a negative breathalyzer test she was skeptical that a judge would buy this argument in the face of a police officer's testimony. This all occurred in a city in another state, so on the day of the court hearing we tensely awaited a phone call from the defense lawyer, fully expecting Monica would lose her case. Surprisingly, the judge was intrigued by the details surrounding HD and dismissed the case. Monica's attorney admitted it was not the outcome she expected, but was very happy she had given it a try. Of course Monica was tremendously relieved and felt justified, even triumphant.

Unpredictable chorea and incoordination can also lead to serious trauma, as was discovered by the individuals in the next set of stories.

27

Broken Bones

As a young adult, Susan already had signs of Huntington disease. She lived by herself in a suburban area and one of her pleasures was to get outside and ride her bike. She roamed the streets and countryside breathing in the fresh Northwest air and waving to passersby. She always wore her helmet. It was never entirely clear what happened to her on that chilly day in March.

Susan and a huge garbage truck met at an intersection and one didn't see the other. She was knocked from her bike, slammed to the road, and her leg was apparently briefly pinned under the truck. Rescue vehicles arrived on the scene and she was transported to the local hospital where X-rays showed nasty fractures of all the major bones in her leg: the thigh bone (femur), and both lower leg bones (tibia and fibula). There was also skin and muscle damage. Two bones required surgery and pinning with metal screws, and that was only the beginning of her complications. Things went from bad to worse. She developed an infection in her lower leg, followed by gangrene, and was transferred to the University Medical Center in Seattle where her leg had to be amputated below the knee.

A lawsuit ensued and attorneys heatedly argued over who was at "fault." I had to testify about her HD and whether it was inappropriate for her to be riding a bike. Although she certainly had a coordination problem, she had never had an accident or previous trouble cycling. Her symptoms of HD did not bother the jury and she won a substantial judgment against the garbage company. Perhaps her diagnosis of HD actually tilted the jury in her favor.

Susan never walked again, and her HD deteriorated rather rapidly. She spent her remaining few years in a nursing home with a private room and personal nurse, compliments of the lawsuit settlement.

■ ■ ■

Bruce Becker's HD made him very agitated and obstreperous. He was quite witty, liked to argue, and tended to be a friendly contrarian. His moods and opinions were unpredictable. One morning he was riding in a county Access bus to a medical appointment. Some unknown aspect of the trip (maybe traffic, maybe the driver, maybe his seat mate, maybe a hallucination) got him very agitated. He suddenly forced open the emergency exit and jumped out onto the freeway with the bus traveling at 50 mph. Not only did this cause a traffic backup for miles, but he broke an arm, two vertebrae in his back, several ribs, and both ankles. His orthopedic hospitalization consumed the next four months, complicated by his contrary behavior of refusing certain medications and usually not participating in rehab. He finally made it back to his adult family home, not the least chastened.

■ ■ ■

Then there was Amanda, who seemed to live in a little world of her own. She was into Buddhism, Zen, vitamin and mineral supplements, and a variety of alternative lifestyles. She existed on a small monthly alimony payment from her ex-husband. She favored long, billowy, Asian clothing and always exuded the aroma of incense. She seemed blithely content with her lonely life and mostly resented people giving her advice.

Amanda rented a room above a garage and had lost interest in personal hygiene. A neighbor complained about Amanda's behavior. A health check report of her apartment from a county inspector described a slovenly atmosphere: dirty, unwashed dishes and clothes mixed with the smell of pot and urine.

At 10 o'clock one night, Amanda was walking alone along an unlit country road and was hit by a pickup truck. She told the emergency responders that she "was looking for the library." Not unlike Bruce Becker, she had broken both legs but also had fractured her pelvis in two places. Also like Bruce, her hospitalization was long and complicated. Multiple X-rays and CT scans identified, unexpectedly, a large tumor looming in her abdomen. One test led to another and she was discovered to have liver cancer. She refused all treatment. "I just want to go home," was all she kept saying. No one wanted to send her back to her miserable room above the garage and so she was discharged to a rehabilitative service in a retirement home. This was after many months in the hospital and she had regained the ability to walk. She liked nothing about her new facility: not the food, not her roommate, not the staff, and not what she feared it might be costing her bank account. One day, she simply disappeared. She had run away and found her way back to her garage. And that is where she stayed. In her own mind the most important thing she could do was hang on to her sense of independence.

▪ ▪ ▪

Susan, Bruce and Amanda show that broken arms and legs and a fractured pelvis can be the "occupational hazards" of having HD. A special case is hitting your head, which, the next chapter shows, is yet another serious risk with HD.

28

A Bump on the Head

Barbara discovered she had taken the wrong bus and needed to make a transfer in busy downtown Seattle. The other riders at the bus stop may have noticed her jerky, twitchy movements, but they didn't bother Barbara. When her bus arrived and the driver opened the door, Barbara tried to climb inside but missed both the step and the handrail. She slipped and fell directly backward, her head hitting the sidewalk with an audible crack. She went limp and was obviously concussed. Someone in the small crowd called 911 on her cellphone and the medics soon appeared. Barbara was taken to the closest hospital emergency department and was wide awake on arrival. An MRI showed bilateral subdural hematomas bleeding into the narrow space between the brain and the skull on both sides of her head. If the blood continued to accumulate there could be compression of the brain and emergency surgery would be required. She was transferred to Harborview Hospital where there were neurosurgeons if she needed them. Her husband was notified and met her in the Harborview ER.

Barbara's hematomas were judged to be relatively small, and X-rays showed no shifting of the brain underneath the clots of blood. She also was awake and talking since her arrival and had no weakness and no headache. She also had no recollection of the bus stop, her fall or of hitting her head. Barbara stayed in the hospital for two days just for careful observation, then went home with her husband. She did not require surgery. The HD caused her to deteriorate further, with increased apathy, less socialization and worse chorea.

Barbara's involuntary movements and poor coordination continued to cause her trouble. She had frequent falls. Once she fell flat on her face, breaking her nose and suffering two black eyes. Another time she fell backward in the shower; she lacerated her scalp and required lots of stitches. She became well recognized in the local hospital ER. Fortunately, repeat MRI scans never showed new hematomas or enlargement of the old ones. Also, Barbara laughed and joked about her falls when told about them because she never remembered them. Her husband thought that she was a bit worse after each fall, but this was difficult to distinguish from the expected slow progression of her disease.

■ ■ ■

On the other side of the county, Hilda's occasional muscle jumps and mild incoordination were not a big problem. She was getting along just fine. She had no trouble managing her household, doing the shopping, or driving around town. One morning, as she was descending the stairs, she missed a step, landed hard on her bottom, and bounced down a few more steps before coming to a stop on the ground floor. She was stunned for a moment, but nothing was broken and she was quickly able to go on about her daily business. Two days later she began to complain of a headache that she had never had before. It wasn't severe, maybe a 5 out of 10 on a pain scale, but it didn't go away. Aspirin and Tylenol were of no help. Two weeks later she still had the headache. She walked out onto her patio and suddenly collapsed onto her barbeque grill and then fell to the floor. She couldn't stand and certainly couldn't walk, but she slowly crawled back inside, found the telephone, and called a friend. Her friend quickly arrived, packed her into her car, and drove her to the local hospital emergency department.

The ER doctor was naturally concerned about Hilda. Although awake and talking, she seemed dazed and a little confused. Furthermore, she was a little weak on the left side. An MRI revealed a large subdural hematoma over the right side of her brain. Neither she nor her family could remember any head injury or even a slight bump on the head, but the fall on the stairs had probably been enough to jar her brain inside her skull. The onset of headache two days later certainly fit that explanation. The local hospital had no neurosurgeon and the decision was made to transfer her to Harborview Hospital in Seattle, the regional trauma center. She still remembers the 50-mile, one-hour ambulance ride on the freeway. She was not worried about the trip but wished someone could get rid of her headache. On arrival at Harborview she had repeat MRI and CT scans. The hematoma was fairly large and was now pushing some of her brain across the midline (Figure 28.1). These images, combined with her mild left-sided weakness, convinced the surgeons that the hematoma needed to be removed. Hilda recalls the calm and informative discussion about what was wrong and what was going to be done. She felt perfectly comfortable and knew she was in good hands. She remembers being rolled into the operating room and then the general anesthesia took over. The surgery was not complicated. Two small holes were drilled in the right side of her skull and the blood was suctioned out.

Hilda was cured. When she woke up in the recovery room her headache was completely gone. Her fatigue and weakness were also gone. She was released the next day. Two years later she is still doing remarkably well at home, knitting, exercising, and taking care of her two grandchildren.

By coincidence, another person with HD was also hospitalized at Harborview while Hilda was there. This woman had set her clothing and hair on fire while smoking a cigarette and putting on makeup while getting ready in the morning. Her movements made this multitasking impossible and exceedingly dangerous. She had to be air

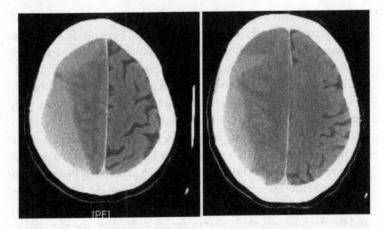

Figure 28.1 ■ CT scans of Hilda's head showing the large collection of blood (subdural hematoma) overlying and compressing the right side of her brain; the hematoma had to be surgically removed. Note that radiologists reverse right and left when printing these images. (With permission of the patient.)

evacuated from Eastern Washington, over the Cascade Mountains, to Seattle and admitted to the Harborview Burn Unit. Her life was saved, but she had disfiguring burns of her scalp, face and arms. For the same reasons that persons like Barbara and Hilda fall and hit their heads, it is well recognized that persons with HD do not do well around fire, especially stoves, ovens and cigarettes. The mixture of poor judgment with impaired coordination and sudden jerky movements can be toxic in these situations. Fires in couches, chairs and beds have led to serious disasters. Coincidentally, Woody Guthrie's life was marred more than once by fires, both during his childhood and as an adult. The cause of these fires was never entirely determined, but it would not be a surprise if they were related to the HD symptoms in his mother and himself.

Anyone who is hit hard enough on the head can develop a subdural hematoma. What is worrisome about HD is that persons with this disease are at a greatly increased risk for subdural hematomas, for two reasons. First, because of involuntary movements and poor coordination they frequently hit their head. Second, as the HD disease progresses there is general shrinkage and atrophy of the brain. This enlarges the spaces between the brain, its covering (the dura), and the skull and may stretch the veins in that area. Even a slight bump on the head can start the bleeding into the subdural space, the clot enlarges, and the damage begins.

29

Impulse Control

The following article appeared in the *Seattle Times* (quoted with permission) under the headline *Court Lets Alleged Flasher Stay Free Despite 10 Arrests*[1]:

Neighbors, prosecutors, social workers a judge and even Jesse Newsom's own lawyers are frustrated. Ten times in the past year he has been charged with indecent exposure, often after allegedly dropping his pants in an apartment window overlooking the swimming pool at the apartment complex where he lives. Each time he was jailed and taken to court, only to be released as incompetent to stand trial but not deranged enough to be committed to a mental institution.

Newsom, 53 has Huntington's chorea, a degenerative disease that killed his mother and sister and has seriously impaired his motor skills and thought processes. He is seized by uncontrollable tics and jerks. The disease also has been blamed for his dementia.

A Prosecutor cited police reports indicating that Newsom's behavior has become more brazen in recent months. "There is nothing more frustrating," he said. "Do we need to wait for a felony, for a victim, until we act? If we know somebody's mentally unstable, let's take them off the streets." Municipal judges don't have authority to lock someone up on mental health grounds, so unless that person commits a felony, or mental-health officials seek a civil commitment, they have no choice but to release him.

At a recent civil-commitment hearing, a court commissioner ruled that Newsom posed no immediate threat to himself or others and thus could remain free. In a recent report, Dr. Frederick Smith determined Newsom was competent while in jail but unable to comprehend the nature, consequences or wrongfulness of his acts. Newsom, who lives on a disability pension, denied in court last week that he was a danger. "I haven't hurt anyone," he testified. Newsom has refused voluntary commitment. When the Municipal Court Judge ordered another evaluation, he told her, "You're wasting my time and yours, your honor."

Neighbors, including a woman who said Newsom exposed himself to her 5-year-old stepdaughter, want him gone. "Our biggest concern is all the children who live around here," she said. "It's harmful. It's not physical, but I don't want my daughter seeing that. It's ridiculous." Several residents of the apartments say management should have him evicted. A manager would not comment. A lawyer for Newsom said he would be best served by commitment. Western State Hospital has a specific ward for people with his disease, she said.

Jesse Newsom's mother died at Western State Hospital in her 60s with a diagnosis of HD. His older brother also had HD and committed suicide. Jesse never married and had no children. He had a positive genetic test for HD and, just as stated in the newspaper article, he was "seized by uncontrollable tics and jerks." He did not go to Western State Hospital. He was ordered to be followed by a psychiatrist and placed on an antipsychotic medication for both his behavior and his movements. Three years after this article appeared he was in an adult care home, barely able to walk or talk. He died three years later.

I have seen three other men with HD who have been arrested for exposure or child abuse. I would not claim that HD caused their specific type of abnormal behavior. The vast majority of persons with HD are not flashers or child abusers. However, comparing Jesse with Johnny, the compulsive thief in Chapter 4, George, the unexpected killer in Chapter 8, and Ward Wilson in Chapter 19, who erased his family's savings with the purchase of an expensive boat, a theme is clearly evident. Impulsivity, disinhibition and lack of social control are common behavioral characteristics of HD. What is not known is why these behaviors play out as sexual in some persons, violence in others, and compulsive gambling and repetitive behaviors or addictions in still others. What is known is that there are regions in the brain that function as controls, monitors or regulators of impulsive behavior. These regions are present in the frontal lobes, and their connections go to the basal ganglia deeper in the brain. These are exactly the areas damaged in HD.

This type of brain disruption and dysregulation of impulses is not specific to HD and is seen in several other neurodegenerative diseases, including frontotemporal dementia (FTD), schizophrenia, and even Parkinson disease. Thus, it is safe to say that HD is a contributing factor to these irregular behaviors, and treatment of these symptoms, though only partially effective, may help decrease their recurrence. Of course, the patients must take their medications and show up for their therapy. All too often they do not.

The lack of impulse control in persons with HD may have some connection to the obsessive-compulsive symptoms that also frequently occur. An *obsession* is a preoccupation with a fixed idea, a *compulsion* is an irresistible impulse to act and to act repetitively. Henry Burger had an obsession that his hands were always dirty. He had a compulsion to continually wash them and scrub them. During one hospitalization he wandered the ward constantly, rubbing his hands with a small wooden brush that had hard, stiff fibers. We would inspect his hands, have him look at them, and tell him they seemed perfectly clean to us. He wouldn't buy it. To Henry his hands were never clean. He was scraping off skin and causing bleeding. We were at least able to convince him to use a softer brush.

Ernest Morgan had an obsession that he was always constipated. This inflexible idea resulted in two compulsive activities. First, he spent hours sitting on the toilet, worried and complaining that there was no bowel action. Second, he drank huge amounts of water, hoping to cleanse his intestines. He once drank so much water that he diluted the electrolytes in his blood. This drove his serum sodium level so low that he became weak, faint and very confused. He required hospitalization to limit his fluid intake and actually infuse some sodium back into his body with an IV drip. He had overdosed on water!

The obsessive-compulsive behaviors of Henry and Ernest went on for months. Eventually, their activities slowly tapered and ended. It seemed that, as the disease progressed, this lack of control over their behavior regressed and was replaced with apathy and inactivity. Whatever the cause of this change, the effect was a relief to their caregivers.

Compulsive behavior overlaps with addictive behavior, and drug and alcohol addiction often occurs in HD, as we will see in the brothers described next with the "reservation blues."

Reference

1. Associated Press. Court lets alleged flasher stay free despite 10 arrests. *Seattle Times*, September 21, 1997, B3.

30

Reservation Blues

The combination of Huntington disease with limited community resources can have distressing consequences. One of the many places we have seen this unfortunate combination unfold is on a Native American reservation.

Johnny and Jerry Greyeagle belong to one of the many small Native American tribes that populate the Pacific Northwest. The family lore is that the brothers' great-grandfather was a white man who had HD and married into the family. Their mother and grandmother both eventually died with the disease. Although Johnny and Jerry are two years apart in age, their stories are so nearly the same that we continually think of them as twins. Growing up on the reservation, they had the double misfortune of being burdened by a mother with HD and a father with severe alcoholism. They loved playing basketball, using a hoop in the dirt driveway of their home. Their mother's coordination became so poor that more than once she crushed the hoop pulling into the driveway. Not long after that she was admitted to a nursing home and died in the same facility where her mother had died. Meanwhile, in an alcoholic rage, the boys' father set fire to their house. The brothers survived, but Jerry was badly burned. Soon thereafter, their father disappeared.

The boys attended a local public school but had little interest in schoolwork. They loved playing basketball, and Johnny became an accomplished weightlifter and boxer. They quit school when Johnny was a junior and Jerry was a freshman. Johnny tried to make a living as a boxer; his ring name was "Warrior." He next tried being a diver for oysters and geoducks (a large member of the clam family that is considered a delicacy in Japan). Jerry tried being a commercial salmon fisherman. None of these jobs lasted for long and their lives became a series of odd jobs in various grocery stores and 7-11s.

The brothers were very attached to each other and became inseparable. They had girlfriends and each produced a child, but never married. Unfortunately, like several other family members, they both became alcoholics. Public intoxication, fist fights and shoplifting led to a long list of interactions with the police and frequent, though brief, stints in jail.

Because of their complicated and erratic behaviors it was difficult to know exactly when they began to show signs of HD. However, they had a tribal mentor named Anthony who had been their basketball coach during adolescence and kept a close eye on them as young adults. When they were around age 30, Anthony became concerned that their coordination was worsening, even when they were not intoxicated. Anthony convinced them to come to our clinic. When we saw them they were quiet but attentive. They asked reasonable questions and freely discussed their social situation, albeit with laconic, short, clipped sentences. They tended to add bits of information to each other's statements. Johnny would say, "I worked in a 7-11 for a while," and Jerry would add, "The pay was lousy." Jerry would say, "I was in jail for fighting and drinking," and Johnny would add, "for two weeks." Jerry had scarring over much of his body from being burned in the old house fire. Both men exhibited clumsiness and mild twitching indicative of early HD. They both requested genetic testing which, not surprisingly, revealed the HD-associated mutation. They had at least two reasons for wanting the genetic testing. One was to decide if their children were at risk for the disease. The other was the hope that having the diagnostic label of HD would increase their chances of getting social and economic resources. They desperately needed resources. Their home was an abandoned trailer on the reservation that had a few chairs and two cots, but no electricity, no running water, and no toilet. They got their water and occasional meals by wandering around the reservation and eliciting assistance from a variety of "aunties," "cousins" and assorted neighbors. They had food stamps and found a nearby public facility for showers. The brothers would sometimes fight and then one would leave the trailer and bum places to sleep from neighbors and relatives for weeks at a time. Anthony and other tribal members were doing all they could to help, but social and financial resources were simply very limited.

Over the subsequent years, the brothers have continued to battle alcoholism and have been in and out of jail. They were always cooperative and never intoxicated when we saw them in the clinic. Johnny developed seizures, probably from a combination of HD and old head trauma from boxing. He was seen by our epilepsy specialists and was able to get appropriate anticonvulsant medication. This stopped the seizures, except when he was drunk and forgot to take his meds, which was too often.

Eventually, they became eligible for Social Security Disability and small monthly checks went to an assigned representative payee. These limited funds allowed the brothers to move out of the nearly useless trailer and into a small, ramshackle house on the edge of town. A care worker was able to visit them several days a week and assist with meals and transportation. Their lives have fallen into a somewhat regular, disorganized rhythm. Each week they get $25 in cash, which they quickly spend on beer, malt liquor, cigarettes and cheeseburgers. The money runs out fast and they spend considerable time panhandling on the street. Their movements have worsened, so Johnny is in a wheelchair and Jerry stands next to him. Their chorea and obvious helplessness brings them sympathy and $50–60 on a good day but nothing on a bad day. This is immediately spent on, beer, malt liquor, cigarettes and cheeseburgers. Their seriously progressing disability will certainly require greater help. It is unclear exactly where that help will come from. They adamantly resist any mention of assisted living or nursing home, remembering that those are the places where their mother and grandmother died.

The problem of meager resources for disabled Native Americans in Washington continues unabated. There are no "casino funds" to help the Greyeagle brothers, or other members of their tribe. Social Security Disability and Medicaid provide a frayed safety net, but the limitations are obvious. The brothers are fortunate to have a tribal mentor watching over them, but there is clearly a need for more help. When supportive resources and a social safety net are completely absent, the individual with HD may be ignored and neglected. We will see how this tragic situation can develop, in the next chapter.

31

Is This Negligence?

The woman on the phone said she was in the State Attorney General's office and wanted me to review a Huntington disease case. She said Calvin had been seen in the emergency department (ED) at Tacoma General Hospital and died in a nursing home a few weeks later. The ED called the police because of suspected abuse and negligence. Photographs taken in the ED by the police documented possible negligence at the man's adult family home (AFH). Would I review the records and photographs and give her an opinion?

A few days later I received a large, heavy envelope containing notes from an AFH, medical records from the hospital, and eight color photographs. I did not know Calvin, but I did know his family. He had undergone a genetic test documenting HD and had spent about two years in the AFH, having been in another AFH before that. There were three other men staying with him, disabled by strokes or Alzheimer's.

Calvin was described as liking to smoke, not liking to bathe, and being clumsy and sloppy because of involuntary movements. He had a past history of "aggressive behavior." During his two years at the AFH he went from walking unsteadily with frequent falls to using a wheelchair to becoming completely bed-ridden. Calvin was entering that last stage of HD but without the aid of a personal, devoted caretaker. Apparently, he was seen on three or four occasions in those two years by a general practice physician who increased his antipsychotic medication each time to eventually quite high doses. Mostly, he was being ignored. The notes kept by the AFH documented a slow but steady decrease in weight, from 163 to 93 pounds. There was no mention of his diet or attempts to feed him. One day, the AFH caretaker dropped him off at the hospital ED, said she could no longer care for him, and left.

The photographs taken in the ED were disheartening and revealed a distressing story (Figure 31.1). Calvin had large, oozing bedsores on both buttocks. His legs, arms and abdomen were covered with cuts

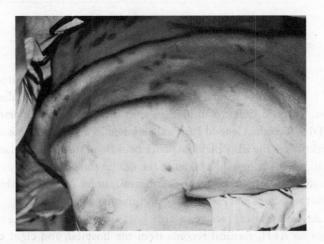

Figure 31.1 ■ Photo taken in the emergency department of Calvin's back showing multiple skin lesions and evidence of weight loss and malnutrition. His head is to the left and his spine is prominent running down his back just above his shoulder blade. (Public Record Document 12-1998-L-0245.)

and bruises and many small round red lesions that looked like cigarette burns. His skin appeared dirty, unwashed and hung loosely over his shoulder and hip bones because of so little muscle and fat underneath. There was no sign of proper nursing care.

Calvin was admitted to the hospital, where he was cleaned, his bedsores dressed, and he was given IV fluids. He communicated with head shakes, eye movements and grunts. His serum protein and albumin levels were low, compatible with chronic malnutrition. After five days of hydration a feeding tube was placed and he was transferred to a nursing home, where he died the following week.

I told the Attorney General's office that there certainly appeared to be negligence in his care. The documented weight loss, the obvious malnutrition, the untreated bedsores, and the dirty, cut, burned skin were obvious indications. She said that was exactly what she thought, but she wanted medical confirmation.

A social service inspector's tour of the AFH listed the following deficiencies:

- Inoperable smoke detector in Calvin's bedroom
- Calvin and roommate were in a bedroom that was too small for double occupancy
- Window in the bedroom was blocked by a bed
- The AFH had allowed health department registration to lapse
- No background check on a nurse who provided services
- Caretaker's husband had unsupervised access to clients and did not hold current CPR and first aid cards and had not completed the fundamentals of caregiving class
- Another person had restrained Calvin with a "bear hug"
- Water temperature in bathroom used by residents was 131°F
- Lapses in recording Calvin's condition and care
- Medication stored in unlocked file cabinet in family room
- Caregivers' prefilled syringes were not properly labeled
- Caregivers did not understand sliding scale for insulin being given to another resident with diabetes
- Calvin not being weighed
- Calvin's diet and meals not documented

Persons with HD are often sitting targets for abuse and neglect. Their movements draw attention to themselves and signal a physical disability. Their confusion and poor judgment often lead them astray and into the hands of charlatans and bullies. Unscrupulous caretakers can take their pensions or Social Security payments and leave out the care. The patients are at the mercy of others.

I called the Attorney General's office a few months later and asked about the outcome of this case. She said the owner of the AFH had lost her certification and was out of business. The patient had no known relatives. No one was pressing further criminal charges.

■ ■ ■

The abuse of vulnerable persons with HD can be even more obvious and alarming. Local police in a town outside of Seattle found a 52-year-old man badly beaten at a community church. He told deputies that he had escaped from a nearby house and that another 37-year-old man was still being held there. When police arrived at the home they found litter and assorted junk scattered around the driveway and yard. They discovered the second victim lying on the ground nearly naked and surrounded by blood. He had broken bones, cuts and burns allegedly sustained from knives and a torch. He was quickly taken to the local ED for treatment and then transferred to Harborview Hospital for more sustained management. It was eventually determined that he suffered from HD and was a member of a large family with the disease that we had followed in our clinic for decades. Two men were arrested, one suspected of leading the abuse and the other an accomplice. They were thought to be stealing their victims' benefit checks, medications and cellphones. The accomplice described his "buddy" beating the victim and keeping him from leaving by taking his clothes and threatening him with a pistol. The lead abuser was described as a heavy drinker who had been arguing with his landlord and causing a general neighborhood disturbance. Thanks to an astute reporter, the local newspaper accurately described the victim as "suffering from Huntington disease, a rare inherited condition that leads to the breakdown of nerve cells in the brain. As the disease progresses it usually results in movements, cognitive and psychiatric disorders according to the Mayo Clinic."[1] Sadly, this was yet another instance of a person with HD being recognized as odd, disabled and vulnerable and then being abused, robbed, and tossed aside.

Reference

1. Binion A. Charges filed in alleged torture case. June 8, 2015. http://archive.kitsapsun.com/news/local/charges-filed-in-alleged-torture-case-ep-1128302793-354673721.html

32

Delusions, Hallucinations and Diabolical Possession

Delusions and hallucinations are considered features of schizophrenia and are often referred to as psychotic manifestations of the disease or psychosis. Delusions may include feelings of persecution, and hallucinations can be auditory or visual. Voices may weave paranoid plots or tell the patients to injure themselves or others. The voices may be unwanted but unavoidable. These characteristics were accurately and powerfully illustrated in the movie *A Beautiful Mind*, based on the true story of John Nash, the brilliant Nobel Laureate in economics who became impaired by recurring delusions and hallucinations.[1] These features are thought to be relatively uncommon in Huntington disease, but they can occur unexpectedly, as we saw in patient David K with his magic watch when we visited Western State

Hospital in Chapter 7. When the psychotic features appear at a young age in persons with HD, before the onset of chorea, it is often argued that the individual actually has two diseases, schizophrenia and HD. However, when the delusions or hallucinations follow the onset of other HD symptoms, there is little question that the psychotic features are a result of the brain degeneration occurring with HD.

Herman Benson illustrates this problem. We saw him in his late 60s, when he came to our clinic with his older sister. He retired in his early 60s from his post office job and lived next door to his sister in a rural community. He had been divorced for many years. His mother had died in her 80s with a diagnosis of late-onset HD. Herman's sister thought that he was getting clumsy and confused, and convinced him to seek genetic testing. He was skeptical of her observations. Nevertheless, he had an adult daughter living elsewhere and decided to obtain genetic testing, for her knowledge and benefit. We met a big man with a firm handshake who was friendly and jocular. He had wispy gray hair and was a little sloppily dressed with a partially tucked-in shirt. He seemed unconcerned about his baggy clothes and, with a wink and smile of genuine pleasure, related that mowing the lawn was his favorite pastime. Jumpy twitches of his arms and face were evident and his hand movements were clumsy. His genetic test showed an abnormal CAG repeat number that was relatively low and fit with his late onset of symptoms. He seemed to be doing reasonably well, and we set up a schedule of annual visits.

Over the next three or four years, Herman's behavior began to deteriorate. He became apathetic, lost interest in caring for himself, and moved in with his sister. He had lost interest in bathing or showering even with considerable prodding from her. He spent most of his time sitting on the couch watching TV, but seemed to pay little attention to the actual content of the programs. Mowing the lawn had previously been one of his favorite activities, which he now completely stopped. In fact, his only physical activity seemed to be once a day, trudging slowly to the end of their long driveway to pick up the mail. Although his involuntary movements had not worsened, his appearance had. He was unshaven, his clothes were dirty, and his body odor was noticeable. He was showing the slow descent into withdrawal and apathy that often happens in HD. Why some persons follow this course while others are agitated and manic has remained a puzzle. In any event, Herman was not a big problem for his sister, other than his lack of cleanliness.

A few years later, things had worsened. He began to ruminate about religion and talk about the battle between good and evil. He decided that the devil had taken up residence inside his body and was telling him to injure other people. He knew the instructions were "bad" but he felt a compulsion to carry them out. He got angry at his sister, threw furniture around, and said the devil was telling him to hurt her. She wisely called 911, and he spent the next few nights in jail. He was referred to a local psychiatrist who admitted him to the hospital and started increasing doses of an antipsychotic medication. Herman calmed down and was able to return home. When we saw him, several weeks later, he remained apathetic and unkempt. He allowed that the devil was still inside him and still telling him to do bad things. He was no longer upset by these instructions and said that he was able to resist. He said resistance was difficult, but he felt he could manage it. And he did. While Satan's voice continued, he seemed able to ignore it. I think the medication was controlling this aspect of his disease even though the inner voice could not be eliminated.

■ ■ ■

We were astonished when a year after meeting Herman, Jason was brought to us because he, too, thought he was possessed by the devil, who was telling him to harm others. Jason was 40 years old, much younger than Herman Benson. His parents had adopted him as a child, and it was known that his biological father had died with HD. Small, intense and cautious, he looked to his parents for answers to anything other than the simplest questions. He was a high school graduate and had had many part-time jobs over the years but was never able to sustain employment. Clumsiness, alcohol addiction, and persistent lack of good judgment led to a diagnosis of HD in his 30s, including a positive genetic test. He had been quite stable and comfortable for several years. But now he said Satan was inside his body and telling him to harm others, including his parents. He seemed angry and volatile and yet he also said he was frightened of the devil and didn't really want to hurt anyone. He agreed to a voluntary inpatient psychiatric hospitalization. Over a period of several weeks, including a premature discharge and quick readmission, he slowly calmed down and was able to return home. Just as with Herman, Satan's voice did not go away and Jason continued to feel possessed. Although he would talk about the devil and the evil instructions, he never acted on them and spent most of his time sitting and reading. At other times he would jump up and try to run out the door, yelling, "I've got to get out of here!" Occasionally, he awoke screaming in the middle of the night, frightened by the devil and wandering wide-eyed into the hall. His father had to grab him, calm him down, and lead him back to bed. Over time, the medication decreased these outbursts and seemed to short-circuit the problems without eliminating them.

The family wondered, "Who was this new person"? He looked like Jason and talked like Jason, but his personality seemed to have dramatically changed.

■ ■ ■

Possession is not always diabolic. In her 30s, Connie insisted that angels in her body had made her pregnant, but she feared a devil might kill her baby. She refused to accept the fact that she actually was not pregnant. After a period of months, this delusion slowly faded.

■ ■ ■

In the disorganized HD brain, the devil may be perceived as possessing someone else. Jacob was yet another man we saw who became hyperreligious and thought Satan was inside his wife and son. The devil was instructing them to plot against Jacob, and he was convinced that he needed to injure them to drive the devil away. This paranoia was dangerous, but since he had not actually injured anyone (yet), he could not be hospitalized against his will, and he refused to go voluntarily. In our clinic it took a series of diplomatic and intense conversations with him, along with three potent drugs (which he was surprisingly willing to take), to eventually get him stabilized.

■ ■ ■

Ben Simon was more tuned into contemporary culture. He was a middle-aged man with the typical symptoms of HD that included mild involuntary movements, apathy, and fairly prominent lack of awareness regarding his movement and behavior problems. He had a caring and supportive wife. Unfortunately, after a few years of regular attendance, he completely stopped coming to the clinic. By phone his wife related that he had become progressively suspicious, frankly para-noid, and angry. They lived in a rural area with no close neighbors. His wife became frightened, left him alone in the house, and moved into a neighbor's house about a half-mile away. She said that he stopped bathing, stopped shaving, and pretty much stopped talking. He cov-ered all the windows with aluminum foil to prevent radiation and radio waves from entering the house. His wife developed the habit of driving to the house, quietly leaving a bag of groceries on the porch and then quickly departing. She said she once sat in her car, perhaps a hundred yards away, and eventually saw him open the door, retrieve the groceries, and disappear back into the house. He had grown a long beard and was stumbling. She was also refilling his antidepres-sant medication and leaving the refills on the porch along with the groceries. She said he would sometimes put the empty pill bottle back on the porch and appeared to be taking the medicine.

However, his medication presented a dilemma. On the one hand, I was glad he was taking it. On the other hand, I could not keep refilling it without seeing him at least once in a while. We devised a medication strategy. I wrote him a prescription for an antipsychotic medication, and his wife left the pill bottle on the porch with the groceries. The hope was that he would take the drug, show some behavioral improve-ment, and be willing to return for a clinic visit. His wife discovered that he did indeed seem to take the new medication. He did not, how-ever, show any sign of improvement. He continued to avoid any type of communication, including her attempts at phone calls and knocking on the door. Eventually, his wife stopped requesting medication refills and we lost all contact with the family. We never really learned how his story ended. It has been many years, and I suspect he is no longer with us.

My mental image of this unfortunate man reminds me of the reclusive Howard Hughes, with his scruffy long beard, uncut fingernails, and his compulsive washing and wiping of doorknobs and faucets. He avoided contact with the outside world. Of course, unlike Ben Simon, Hughes had a millionaire's penthouse in Las Vegas. If he took medication, which I doubt, I always envisioned his chauffeur leaving the bottle on his door step.

■ ■ ■

The delusions in HD are not always diabolical or frightening; they can have a comforting and reassuring aspect. When Carolyn (whom we met in Chapter 12, doing hi-fives) was in a nursing home, in a fairly advanced stage of HD, she was in a wheelchair but still able to carry on a conversation. She had been married 20 years before, but that abusive relationship had ended long ago. One day, with a sly smile and in a low voice to her visiting sister she said, "I got married yesterday." Her sister was taken aback, but being used to Carolyn's frequent mind games responded, "Oh, Really? To who?" Carolyn replied, "To Carlos." Ruth knew that Carlos was the young, good-looking nursing assistant that was very popular with all the residents. She thought at least Carolyn had good taste in her little delusion. Although Carlos was never aware of his matrimonial attachment to Carolyn, she insisted for the remainder of her life that she had a new husband. She would sometimes ask Ruth to take her jacket or pillow to her husband as a gift. Ruth played along with the game, which made Carolyn very happy. The downside was that when she was being transported to a doctor's appointment she would have a screaming panic attack because she thought she was being separated from Carlos.

Things became even more complicated when Carolyn left the facility and moved back into the home of her sister, who was a nurse and could provide her with excellent care. Carolyn decided that she had a baby and talked constantly about the new addition to her family. She would sometimes "find the baby was missing" and cry in despair that someone had taken her baby away. Eventually, Ruth gave her two baby dolls that were kept in a makeshift bassinet by her bed. She loved them, cared for them, and sometimes fell asleep with them in her own bed. She began insisting that she was 18 years old. When her next birthday rolled around she was quite consistent in telling everyone that she was turning 19. For birthday presents she asked for a purple bra and blue jeans. Clearly, her delusions were carrying her back to a younger, happier time.

■ ■ ■

In terms of mental health research, it should be a tantalizing clue that a small but important minority of persons with HD have symptoms so similar to those of schizophrenia. In my experience with HD, there can be quite complex delusions and even auditory hallucinations, just as can be seen in schizophrenia. After decades of research, there is still little known about the biology of schizophrenia. Much more is known about HD, even though it is a far less common disease. The connections between the caudate nucleus of the brain and the frontal lobes are severely disrupted in HD, and something like this must also be happening in schizophrenia. It is important to recognize that both are brain diseases and both cause mental illness. The behavioral aberrations of both HD and schizophrenia can be obvious to those around them. On the other hand, subtle mental changes may not be obvious initially, and the individual slowly loses her or his grip on seemingly simple daily activities, as we shall see in the next chapter.

Reference

1. Nasar S. *A Beautiful Mind*. Simon & Schuster, New York, 1998.

33

The Downward Spiral

Maria Mendoza was pleased with how her life was moving forward in the right direction. She had been born and raised in Argentina, with an excellent education and training in biomedical science. She moved to California at age 22 and got a laboratory technician position in the biotech industry. After a few years she married a handsome, slightly older, successful Argentine businessman living in San Diego. The only burden she seemed to carry was the knowledge that her mother had died with Huntington disease and she had a brother back in her hometown already affected with symptoms. She and her husband decided that she should get tested because they wanted to have a child. Her genetic test revealed the mutation for HD, but she felt fine and had no symptoms. At age 28 she found herself pregnant and decided to have prenatal diagnosis of the baby. The amniocentesis proceeded without difficulty and, joy of joys, the baby was a girl and did not have the genetic abnormality associated with HD. Her daughter would never develop HD.

Maria's husband changed jobs so they moved to Seattle, but she was unable to find employment in biotech. She was good at math and secured an accounting position with a local bank. She was 30 years old when she first appeared in our clinic with her two-year-old daughter, Isabella. "Just checking in with Huntington experts," she said. Maria seemed to have excessive nervous energy, her eyes constantly darting around the room. Although her English was quite good, her conversation wandered and we had trouble keeping her focused. Perhaps tellingly, her husband had not come with her.

The next time we saw Maria she had lost her job with the bank. She said it was because of "downsizing." A supervisor told our social worker that Maria was making too many computational mistakes.

By her next visit to our clinic, Maria still had not found a replacement job and her husband was divorcing her. He had stayed distant from us and from her problem with HD. Not only had he never come to the clinic with her, we had never seen him or had a conversation with him. Now his company was moving him to Virginia, and he was leaving Maria with a small alimony. Little Isabella was now five and there had been no custody battle. Her career-focused father did not want the "burden" of raising his daughter, and Maria was delighted to retain custody.

As the years passed, events continued to deteriorate for the little family of mother and daughter. Maria got a job at a different bank, but she was quickly fired after three weeks. She had developed quite evident chorea with twitches of her hands and body and stumbling when she walked. Her mind wandered and she had trouble keeping track of simple details like the time of scheduled appointments or the payment of household bills. She was still driving but had two non-injury fender-bender accidents. Of course, "It was the other driver's fault." Isabella was now eight years old, in third grade, a bright girl and doing well in school. A neighbor had children that Isabella enjoyed playing with.

We began to have long conversations with this neighbor. She adored Isabella and was happy to have her play in her house. However, she was concerned that Isabella often did not want to leave at the end of playtime and return to her own home. The neighbor realized that Maria was seriously disabled, and she understood the implications of HD. She made several trips to Maria's house and made important discoveries. First, almost all the cooking and food preparation was being done by little Isabella. Second, there was essentially no house cleaning and the home was a total mess: dirty clothes, dirty dishes, piles of old magazines and papers, and mouse droppings. No wonder Isabella stayed away as much as she could. Maria seemed unaware of the problems and resented complaints or even suggestions to tidy up. The thoughtful neighbors banded together and hired a professional housekeeper who spent two days setting things back in order. Of course, it was only temporary.

Maria's ex-husband got wind of the situation. He flew out to visit, took one look, and sued to regain child custody. The legal proceeding was fast. Maria's diagnosis of HD was explained in detail to the judge. At age ten, Isabella left to live with her father in Virginia and never saw her mother again.

Maria was now alone. She lost her driver's license, and her credit cards were canceled. She was on three different medications: one for depression, one for her movements, and one for her behavior, but they seemed of little help. She was visited by a social worker but refused all assistance and simply said she wanted to be left alone. She became obsessed with travel. This obsession seemed to be a combination of trying to get away and an attempt to reach her daughter in Virginia. One morning she appeared for a flight at the United Airlines counter at Seattle Tacoma International Airport. When asked for her ticket, she produced a schedule she had printed of a United flight from Seattle to New York. She didn't seem to understand that producing the schedule was not enough to get her a seat on the plane. The agent was baffled by her behavior but kept explaining it was not going to work. Maria had a temper tantrum—screaming, yelling, tearing up papers, and throwing any objects she could get her hands on. The agent called the airport police, who were finally able to restrain her, calm her down, and send her home.

A few weeks later she again called a taxi to take her to the airport. Carrying two suitcases, she met the cab in front of her house. Because of her disheveled appearance, involuntary movements and confusion, the driver became suspicious. He demanded evidence that she could pay for the $50 trip. She produced a credit card and he discovered it had expired. The only cash she could show was a $5 bill. The driver hopped back into his cab and drove off, leaving Maria standing helplessly in her driveway with her two pieces of luggage, confused, forlorn and alone. The poet Robert Lowell, who knew depression only too well, would say Maria was being overwhelmed by a "landslide of sorrow."

Months later, she appeared at a bus station demanding a ride without any ability to pay. An argument ensued and she again flew into a rage. Screaming at everyone around her, she fought off any attempts to move her outside. The station agent called 911. Medics arrived rather than the police. This was fortunate, because it would have been a mistake to arrest her and toss her in jail. Three medics restrained her and took her to the emergency department at Harborview Hospital. The ED personnel eventually discovered her identity and diagnosis of HD. At first she seemed to consent to a voluntary hospital admission, but later adamantly refused. She remained agitated and belligerent, resisting help and flailing at anyone who came near. A decision was finally made to involuntarily commit her to the locked inpatient psychiatry ward. She was considered "gravely impaired" and the on-call designated mental health professional (MHP) agreed. This was a lucky turn of events, because the MHPs do not always agree with the need for involuntary commitment and such patients may end up back out on the street.

In the hospital, Maria was convinced to take some fairly powerful antipsychotic and tranquilizing medications. She finally calmed down and became more cooperative. By this time, the court had appointed a designated power of attorney who knew her past behavior and was aware of her miserable home situation. Efforts were focused on finding an adult family home that would accept her. This was difficult because of her obvious history of agitated aggressive behavior. A caretaker was eventually found who was willing to take her on, and she was moved into that facility. A major concern, however, was that she might try to run away.

Then, there was one of those unexpected "deus ex machina" moments: an uncle from Argentina appeared on the scene. Her family had heard rumors of Maria's problems and sent Uncle Ignacio to investigate. He met with Maria, her designated power of attorney, and her former neighbors. Amazingly, the family decided to bring Maria back to Argentina and care for her in her final years. Ironically, this turn of events provided the magic plane trip that she had been searching for, taking her away from her misery and back to her home.

■ ■ ■

Stories like Maria's are sadly reminiscent of Dante's slow circular descent into the darkness of the Inferno. Something more is lost each time the person with HD follows a bend on the downward spiral. First a car. Then a job. Then a credit card. Then a house. Then a marriage. Sometimes a child. There is always a hope that some combination of family and community will provide the resources to interrupt the downward spiral. There are successes and failures. Motivation, time, money, facilities and concerned citizens are the requirements, but they are not always there. As a community, we need to do better. Had her distant family not intervened, Maria would most likely have had progressively inadequate help that would have eventually failed her.

Maria disappeared from our view, so we did not follow the last years of her life. The last person with HD described in this section, whom we will meet in the next chapter, remained our patient through the final stages of his disease.

34

A Visit to Willow Park

I drove to the Willow Park retirement community to see Harold. Willow Park is a collection of buildings for retired persons on the west side of King County overlooking Puget Sound. It provides all levels of care: independent apartments and houses, assisted living, advanced nursing care, and a memory unit for persons with dementia. The three- and four-story brick buildings are surrounded by rhododendrons and azaleas. It was the waning days of winter, so the plants had not yet blossomed and their leaves were dark green and edged with brown. Two lovely large willow trees flanked the entrance to the main building. Harold resided on the fourth floor, where his well-to-do family had rented a private room for him and provided one-on-one nursing care 24 hours a day, 7 days a week.

I took the elevator to the fourth floor, walked to the end of the dimly lit hall, and was greeted with a smile at the door by Sofia, Harold's personal nurse's aide. Sofia was a meticulous and dedicated worker with a continually upbeat attitude. Harold was 54 years old and had been a college-educated, successful businessman. I had known him for 10 years since his family brought him to our clinic with twitches and poor coordination reminiscent of those that had occurred much later in life in his father. In retrospect, the family thought Harold had probably had symptoms in his 30s. He eventually had to quit his job because of poor concentration, increasing errors and clumsiness. Four years ago he was in a wheelchair with difficult-to-control movements and slurred speech that made him almost unintelligible. Now he had been completely confined to a bed for more than two years. His neat, clean room had a gorgeous view of the distant snowcapped Olympic Mountains. A television was playing, but the sound had been turned off and actors and actresses in a soap opera flickered silently across the screen. Harold gave no indication of seeing either the lovely view or the TV.

Sofia referred to Harold as "her buddy" and chatted to him constantly as she busied around and cared for his every need. With her impressive strength and energy she turned him, bathed and fed him, oiled and powdered his skin and changed his diaper. She told me how he would respond to her and assist in his care. She said that he would sometimes laugh at her little jokes and ask for changes of the TV channel. I think this personal connection for Sofia was very important to her work ethic and her ability to provide exceptional care. Nevertheless, it had been two years since I had witnessed anything I would call volitional activity on Harold's part. He occasionally moaned or groaned spontaneously when he was moved. However, he had no speech of any kind. I could not get him to follow any simple instructions. Open your mouth: nothing. Stick out your tongue: nothing. Close your eyes: nothing. Move your eyes: nothing. Squeeze my fingers: nothing. He had once been a 6'3", 200 pound athlete. Now he was thin and gaunt, had probably lost 30 pounds in the past four years. He lay in bed with his eyes open and sometimes moved them from side to side, but I could not get him to follow my fingers, my flashlight, or Sofia as she moved around the room. His involuntary movements had disappeared. His arms and legs were now quite stiff and he rarely moved them himself. When I tapped his arms or knees with my reflex hammer his limbs were exceedingly jumpy. Thanks to Sofia, his skin was warm and clean and there was not the slightest hint of a bed sore. Many persons with HD maintain some cognitive abilities even in the late stages of the disease. They can follow commands, answer questions, and recognize family. Others seem to lose all those intellectual functions and one is hard-pressed to tease out any interaction with the outside world. Harold seemed to be one of those whose mental functioning was completely lost.

Harold was still alive because of his superb nursing care and his surprising ability to still chew and swallow food. Although Sofia would probably disagree, the man I met 10 years ago was no longer in the shell of that body. His personality, his character, the Harold we once knew, was gone. I think his wife and son and daughter agreed. They rarely visited. It was just too painful for them. I thanked Sofia once again for her superb nursing care and left Harold behind in Willow Park.

Many, if not most, families with HD have seen or heard detailed descriptions of people like Harold. This is what can await at the end of the HD tunnel. This is the end stage of HD. This is what they fear.

PART V

Summing Up

The preceding chapters have made abundantly clear the traumatic and sometimes ruinous havoc Huntington disease can trigger in a family. It is no surprise that the disease has been a source of medical fascination for more than a century and a focus of intense scientific research for four decades. Although the research has often seemed frustratingly slow, it has actually been making steady progress. A "cure" for HD is not yet in hand, but the final chapter will indicate how the future heralds better days ahead for the world of HD.

35

Summing Up: "Can You Help Me?"

L et us return to the question posed in Chapter 4 by Johnny Cooper from his cell in the Walla Walla Penitentiary: "Can you help me?" Naturally, this is the question asked of doctors by all their patients. The traditional guidelines for physicians stretching back to Hippocrates are to "relieve suffering and do no harm." The answer to Johnny's question is: sometimes we can help a great deal, sometimes we can only help a little, and sometimes we just muddle through as best we can, navigating our way between suffering and harm.

To be specific about Huntington disease, there are certainly treatments that help. From my personal experience, most persons with HD eventually develop some degree of involuntary movements that can be mild, moderate or severe. In a subgroup of HD patients, the chorea is the most disabling aspect of the disease. There are several medications that can improve chorea, with results varying from minimal to dramatic. In another small percentage of patients there is clumsiness and incoordination, above and beyond the chorea, that is probably caused by pathology in the cerebellum and the white matter tracts of the brain. (The cerebellum manages the coordination of body movements and white matter tracts carry nerve cell messages from one part of the brain to another.) This incoordination combined with the involuntary movements can be very disabling and not very amendable to treatment. Another small subset of patients do surprisingly well with their disease and require little in the way of therapy. They are generally the persons with relatively small, albeit abnormal, CAG repeat expansions in the *HTT* gene.

This leaves the majority of people with HD, who are primarily disabled by the behavioral and cognitive manifestations of the disease. The chapters in this book provide numerous examples of these problems that could fall under the umbrella term of *mental illness* and, like all mental illnesses, these symptoms are caused by an underlying brain dysfunction. The list of behavioral and cognitive disabilities associated with HD is long and daunting: agitation, aggression, apathy, impulsivity/disinhibition, depression, lack of awareness, poor attention span, impaired judgment, obsessive-compulsive syndrome, and delusional thinking. There are dozens of medications that can sometimes ameliorate these symptoms, including antidepressants, antipsychotics, mood stabilizers and tranquilizers. Again, the results vary from minimal to dramatic. Of course, they all also have side effects that vary from no problem, to tolerable, to intolerable.

In addition, there are a number of non-medication approaches to both behavioral and physical problems that can be quite valuable. These include psychotherapy, behavioral counseling, speech and swallowing therapy, and physical therapy.

The clinical approach to patients and families with HD has three key components:

(1) *Compassion* for the patients and their problems, no matter how troubling or desperate; over time, compassion may even blossom into empathy.

(2) *Determination* that the problems can be solved, no matter how complex or daunting.

(3) *Patience,* recognizing that time is a factor and success will come in increments.

Finally, perhaps the greatest help for persons with HD is to have a supportive social environment of concerned and empathetic friends and family. As demonstrated in the vignettes in this book, some people with HD have no social support, some have it and lose it, and others have it in strength and permanence. The stress of HD can be nearly overwhelming for spouses, children, parents and siblings. Many people with HD and their families experience the five stages of grief identified by Kübler-Ross: denial, anger, bargaining, depression and acceptance. Not all persons encounter all stages, nor are the stages always experienced in a certain order. Nevertheless, these simple labels effectively capture the emotional trajectory of facing HD. The "acceptance" phase hopefully results in a form of resilience and coping that represents flexible strength—the ability to bend, but not break. Many of the patients with HD and their family members exemplify the Japanese word *gaman,* which roughly translates as "the impressive ability to endure the seemingly unbearable with patience and dignity."

As amply described in this book, families can be overwhelmed by HD. This is especially true when the family member develops behavior that is out of control. While huge state mental institutions can no longer be justified, there remains a need for smaller, focused facilities that can keep a patient safe, calm and redirected. Such individuals may require an admission lasting 30 days or even 3 or 4 months. Today's adult family homes and assisted living facilities are usually woefully inadequate to care for behaviorally disturbed patients. Places providing intense behavior management need highly trained, professional and dedicated staffs, with adequate funding to maintain quality standards. Such facilities are not cheap, but in the long run they are well worth the cost.

Unfortunately, at the present time there is no "cure" for Huntington disease. I put the word *cure* in quotation marks because there are actually different ways to view or define a cure. There is nothing that stops the advance of HD once it has started. There is nothing that slows the pathological progression, although the disease takes different trajectories in different persons. There is nothing that reverses the disease. There is nothing that prevents the onset of the disease. No matter how you view it, there is really no specific treatment for this progressive degenerative brain disease. In other words, no matter how you look at it, there is no "cure."

The good news is that the advances over the past 20 years in understanding the biology of brain diseases has been phenomenal and highly encouraging. In addition to Huntington disease, this impressive research includes that related to Alzheimer's, Parkinson's, FTD, ALS, schizophrenia, and depression. The gene that, when altered, causes HD was identified in 1993. Subsequently, a huge body of knowledge concerning the molecular biology and biochemistry of the disease has been established, yet a specific treatment has not been forthcoming. Nevertheless, the groundwork has been laid to reach this goal. The goal is attainable, and the research should not be slowed. Much of this research is done by the National Institutes of Health (NIH), which requires strong public and legislative support. Private organizations, such as the Hereditary Disease Foundation and the CHDI Foundation, also promote valuable focused research on HD. The research needs to be broad, from A (Alzheimer) to Z (Zika virus–related microcephaly), and deep, from social psychology to molecular biology. The scientific approach to this disease is also international, including important work being done in Canada, the United Kingdom and Germany.

Moving forward, the following is a partial list of research projects focused on treatment of HD that could prove fruitful:

- Development of medications that suppress delusions and violent behavior without inducing lethargy and lack of initiative.
- Better treatments for depression. Such therapy would be of great benefit for mental health far beyond HD.
- A drug that would improve faulty judgment. While this seems like a fantasy and wishful thinking, this impairment

is one of the most serious deficiencies in HD. Such an
approach would require a much better understanding of the
neurophysiology of frontal-lobe executive functions.

- Better understanding of the biochemical and physiological
  determinants of movement and coordination that would lead
  to improved control of chorea, tremor and ataxia. This, in
  turn, would lead to prevention of falls and trauma, enabling
  more independent living.

- Attempts to silence the genetic mutation in HD, building on
  studies already underway. Successful implementation of such
  research would produce astounding possibilities for both
  treatment and prevention of HD and of many other similar
  degenerative brain disorders. If this genetic technology
  actually led to prevention of HD, the overused and much-
  abused terms *astounding, ground-breaking* and *breakthrough*
  would be quite appropriate for this development. Exciting
  clinical trials using this genetic approach are underway at the
  writing of this book.

- Additional therapeutic approaches to HD, such as those
  highlighted by Bates and colleagues[1] and Dickey and
  LaSpada,[2] taking advantage of new knowledge of the
  disease that has been generated over the last two decades.
  This push toward the therapeutic future bodes well for
  the eventual taming of this disease. The recent successful
  genetic treatment of spinal muscular atrophy in children is
  a shining example of a therapeutic triumph over a genetic
  neurodegenerative disease.

For the present, the best immediate resource for the evaluation
and management of patients and families with HD comes from the
Huntington's Disease Society of America (HDSA). This commendable
organization has established more than 40 HD Centers of Excellence
around the country which provide desperately needed assistance for
families dealing with HD. As mentioned earlier, while we search for a
cure, organizations such as HDSA, which are providing hard-to-come
by resources, need our support and encouragement.

As noted before, the genetic abnormality causing HD was discovered in 1993. In those heady days of gene discovery there was considerable enthusiasm among both scientists and families that this would soon lead to major breakthroughs in treatment. Now, more than 20 years later, it has become clear that the path from gene discovery to effective treatments is long and winding. Capitalizing on these scientific achievements is arduous. Incredible mouse models of HD now exist, but moving from mouse to human is difficult and tricky business. Conquering neurodegenerative diseases will require a comprehensive and sustained basic-science approach, in addition to discovery of new pharmaceuticals and treatment trials.

Patience and steady progress should be the mantra for conquering HD; do not expect miracles. Expect slow, steady progress. The motto of a hospital I worked in as a student was: "Every day, in every way, a little better." So it should go with Huntington disease, so that the frustrating and often overwhelming brain disease illustrated in this book will one day disappear.

References

1. Bates GP, Dorsey R, Gusella JF, Hayden MR, Kay C, Leavitt BR, Nance M, Ross CA, Scahill RI, Wetzel R, Wild EJ, Tabrizi SJ. Huntington disease. *Nature Reviews. Disease Primers*, 1:15005, 2015.
2. Dickey AS, LaSpada AR. Therapy development in Huntington disease: from current strategies to emerging opportunities. *American Journal of Medical Genetics*, 176(4):842–861, 2018.

ACKNOWLEDGMENTS

I t has been difficult to wrap my mind around my experience with Huntington disease. The anecdotes and vignettes in this book are an attempt to do just that, but represent only a fraction of an almost overwhelming number of complicated encounters. Over the past 45 years, I have had repeated interactions with more than a thousand Huntington patients from many hundreds of families. I am especially indebted to several members of those families who have shared their perspectives for this book. They include Josh and Joe Andrews, Tim Bittrick, Perry Carrington, Justin Cheverny, Hilde Foreman, Albert and Cathie Gillet, Kathryn Harrild, Cathy Hatch-Daniels, Margaret Hemingsen, Jay Hemphill, Beverly Hertig, Jennifer Jenkins, Connie and Perry Kirschner, George Neilson, Sally Rose, Richard Rosenwald, Kathleen Ruen, Kenneth and Lucia Schubert, Ruth Trembaly, and Holly Wall. Vanessa Perry allowed me to reprint sections of her third-grade class' description of juvenile HD.

Over the years I have worked alongside a wonderful group of volunteers who organized and maintained the Seattle and Pacific Northwest HD support groups. These include Wilma Berman, Katy

Bradley, Jim Bridges, Roger Carnes, Greg Colucci, Merle Denny, Marie Dunn, John and Vicki Early, E.J. Garner, Linda Ingle, David Johnson, Debbie and Joyce Korevaar, Betty and Vicki Kost, Jerry Mickelson, Ted Morgan, Phil Pearson, Jaquie Stock, Vivian Thevik, Liz Webber, and Steve Weil. Dr. Lavonne Goodman has been greatly appreciated as a powerful advocate for HD in the Northwest and nationally.

Social workers have been a crucial factor in providing professional and caring support for the HD families. The pioneering work of Amelia Schultz has already been recognized in the dedication, and she was very capably followed by Catherine Kendall, Donna Ross, Chris Wick, and Susan Reynolds. Jolie VonSuhr organized our important field trip to Western State Hospital.

Several dedicated hard-working nurses have been instrumental in the care of our HD patients, including Hillary Lipe, Brenda Vicars, Brenda McNee-Thorson, and Johna Vickers.

Brenda Vicars and Susan Reynolds deserve special recognition for creating an incredibly hard-working and effective HD support team at the University of Washington that has benefitted hundreds of families.

Outstanding genetic counselors have helped these families navigate the difficult terrain of genetic counseling and testing. These marvelous people include Robin Bennett, Corrie Smith, Sarah Mickelson, Mercy Laurino, Susie Ball, Cindy Dolan, Lael Hinds, and Lauren Brown.

Debbie Olsen capably coordinated the UW Medical Genetics Clinic and tried to keep us all on schedule.

I am a neurologist, largely because of remarkable mentoring by Drs. Francis King at Dartmouth College and Fred Plum at Cornell Medical College. At the University of Washington, Drs. Phil Swanson and Don Farrell encouraged me to become a clinical neurogeneticist, a specialty that did not exist at the time, and Dr. Arno Motulsky provided me with the opportunity to make that happen. It was in the early pursuit of that career that I began the evaluation, care and management of patients with Huntington disease. Dr. Suman Jayadev is a wonderful neurology colleague who now directs the UW HDSA Center of Excellence. She is ably assisted by Dr. Marie Davis, with her expertise in movement disorders; Dr. Matt Schreiber, who brings his experience in psychiatry; and Dr. Fuki Hisama, director of the UW Medical

Genetic Clinic. Drs. Mark Sumi and Dr. Dirk Keene are outstanding neuropathologists who have worked with me on hundreds of families with neurogenetic diseases.

Lucretia Fishburn in the Attorney General's Office gave me helpful advice.

The Seattle VA Medical Center provided me with the time, space and resources to pursue decades of clinical and research projects. The veteran patients at this facility are very special people cared for by an excellent and highly dedicated staff.

Nationally, the HD community is heavily indebted to Debra Lovecky and the amazing individuals associated with the national office of the Huntington Disease Society of America, including Louise Vetter and George Yohrling.

I have had very helpful conversations with my colleagues in the HD community who have shared so many similar experiences, especially Martha Nance, Vicki Wheelock, Elizabeth Aylward, and Terry Tempkin. These people, as well as Alice and Nancy Wexler, encouraged me to get my memories down on paper.

Sarah Elmore spent many hours typing and retyping the entire manuscript.

Cindy Dolan, Jack Bernard, Marilynn Westerman, Joe Pearl, and Robin Lindley all read the manuscript and provided superb feedback and suggestions.

My brother John, the eternal optimist, will never fully realize how much he influenced me.

The first draft of this book was finished in the spring of 2015. It clearly required an editor and publisher. Fortunately, I found Craig Panner, my editor at Oxford University Press, who had the vision to see the value of this project and the experience to keep me focused.

Finally, I would have never made it intact through all these years without the incredible support and grounding provided by my wife, Ros. She helps me integrate the science and the arts. Thank you so very much.

Genetic Testing for Huntington Disease

The genetic test result is not black and white, all or nothing. The gene (*HTT*) associated with Huntington disease has a normal form that is present in all of us. This normal form of the gene codes for a protein that is important for brain cell function. The genetic test for HD is based on determining the number of pieces of DNA in a certain region of this gene. The region is called a *CAG repeat*, referring to the three chemicals (cytosine, adenine, and guanine) linked in a row in the DNA. Although this stretch of DNA is relatively stable, it does have the potential to expand or contract. It normally contains about 10–20 pieces of DNA. When the region enlarges or expands it is called

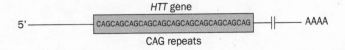

HD is caused by a CAG repeat expansion in the *huntingtin* gene on chromosome 4p

HTT gene

5'———————[CAGCAGCAGCAGCAGCAGCAGCAGCAGCAGCAGCAG]—||—— AAAA

CAG repeats

Number of CAG Repeats
Normal: 11–27
Unstable Intermediate: 28–34
Decreased Penetrance: 35–39
Full Penetrance: 40+
Juvenile: 60+

Figure A.1 ■ The gene (*HTT*) that codes for the protein (called huntingtin) involved in Huntington disease (HD) resides on the short arm (p) of human chromosome 4 and codes for a protein containing 3,144 amino acids. This cartoon shows only the initial portion of the gene, illustrating the region carrying the CAG repeats. The three letters indicate three chemical nucleotides (C for cystine, A for adenine, G for guanine) in the DNA molecule. Expansion of the CAG region of this gene (indicated by the blue box) causes HD when it contains more than 39 CAG repeats. *Full penetrance* means that anyone having an expansion in this range will develop symptoms of the disease during a normal lifespan. *Decreased penetrance* means the expansion is "abnormal" but the individual may or may not develop symptoms of the disease. Persons with an expansion in the unstable intermediate range are not expected to develop symptons of HD, but because the expansion is unstable when transmitted to their offspring, their children have a small risk of inheriting a larger expansion. CAG expansions larger than 60 are often associated with onset before the age of 20 (juvenile HD). None of these numbers are absolute indicators of disease but represent a gradual scale of overlapping ranges. For example, some juvenile-onset children have CAG expansions less than 60.

a *CAG repeat expansion* (Figure A.1). It is the size of this repeat region that serves as the basis of the genetic test for HD.

• When this CAG repeat expands to 40 or greater the individual is destined to develop symptoms of HD if he or she lives a normal lifespan, although the exact age of onset cannot be predicted. This is called the *range of full penetrance*.

- If the expansion is 60 or greater the onset of symptoms is often in childhood (before age 20), so is called *juvenile HD*. When the expansion is greater than 80 the onset may be before age 10.

- An expansion size of 35–39 is problematic, the so-called *range of decreased penetrance*. Some persons with an expansion in this range develop symptoms of HD and others do not. The age of symptom onset in this range is often after 60. Nevertheless, each of their children, male or female, is at 50% risk for inheriting the expansion, and it may enlarge when it is transmitted to them.

- Expansions in the range 27–34 (the indeterminate or intermediate range) are rarely, if ever, associated with symptoms of the disease, but are somewhat unstable and may rarely enlarge into a more abnormal range when passed on to a child.

- All of these expansion size numbers and their consequences are important but inexact estimates. A single repeat number such as 43, although abnormal, cannot predict an exact age of onset of symptoms.

- It is also important to note that the genetic test result does not indicate the type or severity of symptoms the individual may develop.

The size of the DNA repeat varies in the general population, usually being somewhat smaller in Asians and Black Africans, which apparently explains why HD is less common in these groups. That is, the likelihood that the repeat will expand into a disease range is lessened.

Changes in the chemical sequence of DNA are called *variants*. When the change produces an abnormality so severe that it is directly associated with a disease, it is called a *pathogenic variant*. These pathogenic variants have traditionally been called *mutations*. This older term (*mutation*) is often used in this book to refer to the pathogenic variant in the *HTT* gene associated with HD.

The terms *positive* and *negative* for the genetic test result are often used by healthcare providers. "Positive" in this context means "abnormal," that is, the CAG repeat has expanded into the range associated with symptoms, or the eventual development of symptoms, of Huntington disease (e.g., 40 or more). "Negative" means a CAG expansion size not associated with symptoms (e.g., less than 28). This wording leaves out expansion sizes between 28 and 40 and does not indicate the often complex interpretation of the test results, which always requires careful explanation. For simplicity, the term *positive* is sometimes used in this book to refer to the genetic test result, but the reader should remember that the actual result is more complicated than a simple "yes" or "no." The various ways in which people may respond to genetic test results are described in Chapter 3.

INDEX

References to figures are denoted by an italicized *f*.

abnormal behavior, 78–79
abuse and neglect, 193
  Attorney General reviewing, 219,
    221, 222
  Calvin (HD) from adult family
    home (AFH), 219–21
  deficiencies in social service
    report, 221
  persons with HD as target for, 222–23
  photograph of Calvin's back with
    skin lesions, 220*f*
acceptance, 247
adoption
  Catholic agency, 172–73
  families with HD, 136
  Janet's desire for children, 167–70
  Judge, 173
  VanDuser's adopting daughter Vicki
    (HD), 171–76
  see also VanDuser, William and Evelyn
adult care home/adult family home,
    46–47, 176, 188, 202
  Attorney General reviewing, 219,
    221, 222
  Bailey Boushay House, 188–90,
    191–92
  Calvin (HD) and neglect in, 219–21
  deficiencies in social service
    report, 221
Air Force, 187–88

alcohol
  abuse of, 40, 41, 80–81
  addiction, 227–28
  attraction to, 98
  compulsive behavior and, 214
  drugs and, 40, 43, 80–81, 214
alcoholism, 3, 215–16, 217
Allen, Ron, 140–41
alpha synuclein, PD, 17
ALS. *See* amyotrophic lateral
    sclerosis (ALS)
Alzheimer, Alois, 13–14
Alzheimer disease, x, 6, 23, 104,
    219–20, 248
  amygdala and, 66–67
  brain pathology in, 13–14
  comparing HD with, 13–14
  dementia in, 13–14, 53–54
  familial early-onset AD, 14, 59
  progression of, 12
  rare form of inherited, 61–62
  thousand mile stare, 14
American Psychosis (Torrey), 58
amniocentesis, 233–34
amygdala, 66–67, 80–81
amyloid and tau, AD proteins, 17
amyotrophic lateral sclerosis (ALS),
    16, 47–48
  ice-bucket challenge, 100
  support group, 101

anosia, 114–15

anosognosia, 114–15

antidepressants, 18, 25, 106, 109–10, 145, 146, 158, 229, 246

antipsychotic medication, 68–69

antisocial personality disorder associated with callous/ unemotional traits, 80–81

apathy, 155

Arizona prison system, 144–45

Army, 165–66

assisted living, 98, 99, 138, 139

assisted suicide, 47–48, 139–40

asylum(s)

deinstitutionalization, 57–58

embarrassment of confinement, 51

historical background of "insane." 52–53

morgue at Western State Hospital (WSH), 59–62

treatment in, 53–57

attention deficit hyperactivity-autism spectrum, 143

auditory hallucinations, schizophrenia, 18–19

autism, ix, 66–67, 143

autopsy, brain removal for research, 60–61, 62

autosomal dominant genetic form

Alzheimer disease (AD), 14

amyotrophic lateral sclerosis (ALS), 16

frontotemporal dementia, 15

Bachman, Brian, 38

arrest for stealing, 49–50

brother Carl, 43–44

deterioration after Carl's death, 44–45

emergency department (ED) and, 46, 48

family members of, 40

genetic testing for, 41–43

intensive care unit (ICU), 49

life in clinic, 49

living environment, 44–45

as male fashion model, 40–41, 42f, 45–46

story of, 39

trouble for, 49–50

Bailey-Boushay House, 188–90, 191–92

Marie and Michael's experience at, 188–92

Michael (HD) and Marie's experience at, 188–92

Tom (HD) and Virginia at, 190, 191–92

basal ganglia, 6, 7f

Bates, GP, 10, 10, 250

A Beautiful Mind (film), 106–7, 225–26

Becker, Bruce, 202, 203

Becker, Chester, 163–64

behavioral counseling, 246

Bellisle, M, 62

Bennett, Tim

ALS and ice-bucket challenge, 100

ALS support group, 101

coping skills, 99–101

double diagnosis of HD and ALS, 101

electromyogram (EMG), 100

HD support group, 100

teaching, 99, 100, 101

Benson, Herman, 226–27

Binion, Andrew, 223

bipolar disorder, 6, 18, 45–46, 155

Bird, Thomas D., 34, 35

Blair, RJR, 81
Blake, Casey, 81
bones. *See* broken bones
bowling, positive attitude, 98
brain
    anatomy for HD, 1
    autopsy for research, 60–61, 62
    biology of disease, 248
    caudate nucleus, 6, 7*f*, 231
    degenerative disease of, ix
    disconnection in, 78–81
    disease, 45–46
    frontal lobes, 231
    medium spiny neurons, 6, 7*f*
    mitochondria of cells, 7
    pathology in AD, 13–14
    striatum of the basal ganglia, 6, 7*f*
The Brain Defense (Davis), 80
Brewer, Monica, 198–99
broken bones
    Amanda and pickup truck
        accident, 202–3
    Bruce Becker jumping from bus,
        202, 203
    occupational hazards of HD, 203
    Susan (HD) in bike accident, 201–2
Brown, Megan, 89–90
Browne, James Crichton, 52
Buddhism, 202–3
bupropion, 146
Burger, Henry, 213–14
Burroughs, Bernie, 157–59
Bus Driver, Metro, 198

CAG (cytosine, adenine and
    guanine) expansion repeats, 5,
    245–46, 255–56
    abnormal, 5, 26, 77–78, 80–81,
    115–16, 151–52, 226

high/large, 66, 128–29, 153, 256*f*
HTT gene, 6, 128, 183, 245–46
intermediate, 6
juvenile HD, 6, 128–29
low/small, 5, 97, 109, 122, 123, 258
reduced penetrance, 6
repeats, 5, 72, 256–57
canary in the mine, HD as, x, 32
Carkeek Park, Seattle, 83, 84*f*, 86
Carr, Carol, 139–40
case histories, x
Catholic adoption agency, 172–73
caudate nucleus, 6, 7*f*
    brain, 231
    Huntington disease, 7*f*
centers of excellence, 249
cerebellar ataxia, 33–34
Changeling (film), 106–7
CHDI Foundation, 248
children with HD
    cover of booklet "Princess in Pink,"
        133*f*, 130
    death of Bobbi, 133–34
    pages of "Princess in Pink," 131–32
    positive approach of teacher,
        129–30, 133
    story of Bobbi, 127–29
    see also juvenile Huntington disease
chorea, 6, 53–54, 113–14
    criminal Dr. Gilmer with, 79–80
    example of "The Smoker", 9
    involuntary movements, 195
    letters with Mr. Cooper
        regarding, 34, 35
    Parkinson disease, 15–16
    variability of, 11–12
chorionic villus sampling, 168
Christmas, holidays and social
    interactions, 178

Cohen, Bruce, 20
Cold Spring Harbor Laboratory, 3
Come and Get It (film), 54–56
comfort object, book as, 68
compassion, 246
compassionate care, 22, 52, 66, 133,
    165, 190
compulsion, 213–14
    Ben Simon and, 229–30
    Howard Hughes, 230
compulsive behavior, 214
compulsive gambling, 213
computed tomography (CT), 6, 203,
    207, 208*f*
conduct disorder, 80–81
Cooper, Johnny, 33–34, 35–36, 245
    compulsive stealing by, 37, 38
    death of mother, 57–58
    interactions after prison, 36–37
    letters with, 34, 35
coping strategies
    ALS support group, 101
    HD support group, 100
    onset of HD, 93
    recognizing happy lives, 94
    suicide, 94
    symptomatic Huntington disease, 93
    Tim Bennett's, 99–101
    unproven remedies, 93
coroner, HD gene testing, 89–90
counseling
    term, 21
    see also genetic testing
Creedmoor Hospital, Queens,
    New York, 53, 54*f*
Creutzfeldt-Jacob disease (CJD),
    degenerative brain disease, 16–17
criminality, 3
Crowe, Russell, 106–7

Crowley, Betty, 117, 118
Cusin, C, 111

dancing, positive attitude, 96–97,
    103–4
Davenport, Charles, 3
Davenport, Jack, 164
Davis, Kevin, 80
death, 21–22, 27, 148. *See also* suicide
"Death with Dignity" Washington state
    law, 47–48
decreased penetrance, 256*f*, 257
Dedman, Bill, 119
delusions, 11–12, 194, 225–26
    Carolyn in nursing home, 230
    denying, 76
    schizophrenia, 18–19
    see also possession
dementia patients, Washington State
    Hospital, 64–65
denial
    case of Mr. Z, 113
    HD diagnosis, 114–15
Department of Motor Vehicles, 198
depression, 6, 8, 13, 21–22, 53–54,
    101–2, 145, 155, 248
    Albert Sullivan, 105–11
    bipolar disorder, 18
    common in HD, 18
    electroconvulsive therapy (ECT)
        and, 145–46
Depression, 121–22
determination, 247
diagnosis
    Betty Crowley unaware of, 117
    Gordon Thomas lacking awareness
        of, 117–19
    Mr. Z disagreeing with, 113
Dickey, AS, 250

disability insurance, 26
disability pension, 212. *See also* Social
    Security Disability
disconnection, brain, 78–81
disinhibition, 80–81, 118, 213
disinhibition associated with brain
    damage, 80
Dix, Dorothea, 52
domestic violence, 80–81
driver's license, 235
driving, 116
driving test, 198
Dukakis, Kitty, 107–8

Eagleton, Thomas, 106–7
Eastern State Hospital, Washington
    state, 69–70f
education
    genetic, 21
    Huntington disease, 21–22
    special, 76
electroconvulsive therapy (ECT), 12,
    53–54, 145–46
    depression and Kitty Dukakis, 107–8
    depression in Albert, 106, 108, 109–11
    machine, 107f
electroencephalogram (EEG), brain, 77
electromyogram (EMG), 100
electroshock, 53–56
    early machine, 71–72
    therapy, 106–7, 145
embarrassment, 160, 51, 193, 196
emergency department (ED), 46, 48
emotional recognition, deficit, 66–67
employment
    Army and Steven Robbins, 165–66
    Ben (HD) and, 182–83
    challenge of staying employed, 161
    engineer Chester Becker, 163–64

filing clerk Jennifer, 165
    symptoms of HD, 136
    teacher Sandra Smith, 161–62
    teacher William Harris, 162–63
    truck driver Jack Davenport, 164
engineering, ceiling railway system for
    transport, 148–49
epilepsy, 128–29, 217
Esquire (magazine), 40–41, 42f
eugenics analysis, 3

family history, choreic, of patient at
    WSH, 69–70f
family life
    downward spiral, 237
    holidays and social
        interactions, 177–78
    Maria Mendoza decline, 233–37
    persons with HD, 135
family members, HD impact on, 139
Farmer, Frances, 54–56, 71–72, 106–7
Federal Interagency Committee on
    Mental Health, 58
Fields, W. C., 154–55
finances
    accountant Leonard Reynolds with
        HD, 156
    Andrew (HD) and VA pension
        system, 151–52
    Bernie Burroughs, 157–59
    Eddie (HD) and homelessness,
        153–54
    symptoms of HD, 136
    Ward Wilson and mania, 154–55
founder effect, 3
Frances (film), 106–7
Freeman, Walter, 54f, 55–57
frontal lobes, brain, 231
frontal lobotomy, 54–56, 71–72

frontotemporal dementia (FTD), 15,
78–79, 213, 248
full penetrance, 256f, 257

Gage, Phineas, 78–79
gaman (Japanese word), 247
general parasis of insane (GPS), 53–54
genetic testing, 114, 233–34
comments from experiences, 23–24,
25, 26–29
common motivation for
exploring, 22
considerations for HD test, 23
coroner request for, 89–90
discovery of HD gene, 92
for Huntington disease (HD),
255–58
Huntington gene and, 4
positive attitude by Mary, 95–96
prenatal, 168, 169
pros and cons of, 41–43
range of test results, 22
reactions to, 30
reasons for, 216–17
results, 5, 258
reviewing for Mr. Z, 115
suicide and, 26–27, 28
survivor guilt, 27–28
Genova, Lisa, 23, 30
George VI (King), 188
Gilmer, Ben, 79–80
Gilmer, Vince, 79–80
Grafton, Sue, 11–12
Grant, Ulysses, 52–53
Greatest Generation, 121–22
Greyeagle, Johnny and Jerry, 215–18
gunshot, suicide by, 159
Guthrie, Woody, 18, 23, 53, 55f, 100,
124, 155, 207–8

hallucinations, 202, 225–26
auditory, 18–19
denying, 76
handwriting illegible, 33–34
Harborview Burn Unit, 207–8
Harborview Hospital, 189–90, 207,
222–23, 236
Harris, William, 162–63
Harvard Law School, 154–55
Hayden, M, 7
head injuries
Barbara's subdural hematomas, 205–6
Hilda after falling down stairs, 206–8
health insurance, 26
Hedges, Phoebe, 1, 6, 4
Hemingway, Ernest, 18
Hereditary Disease Foundation, 248
hereditary neuropathy, 33–34
hippocampus, brain pathology in
AD, 13–14
Hippocrates, 245
hoarding behavior, 181–82
Hoke, Chris, 92
homelessness, 68–71, 153–54,
174, 177–78
horned toad defense, 75–76
hospice, 111, 133–34, 152–53, 165, 176
Hospital Bicetre in Paris, 65–66
HTT gene, 6, 128, 183, 245–46,
255–56, 257
Hughes, Howard, 230
huntingtin gene, 1, 17
Huntington, George, 1, 6, 3, 4
photograph, 2f
Huntington disease (HD), ix–x
behavioral component, 8
brain anatomy of, 6
brief history of, 1
cognitive component, 8

cure lacking, 243, 247–48
description of, ix–ix
discovery of genetic
    abnormality, 250
doctor recognizing in shopper, 195–96
driving by patient with, 116
dual diagnosis of ALS and, 101
education, 21–22
genetic testing for, 255–58
implications, x
intoxication suspected in, 196, 197–99
involuntary movements of, xi, xii, 8
judging when HD begins, 13
juvenile-onset, 66, 93, 128–29
medical context of, 10
migration, 3
motor part of, 8
movement disorder, 8
patients in legal and mental
    healthcare systems, 31–32
research projects, 248–49
severity in United States, 3
symptomatic persons and family
    members in U.S., 3
symptom development by age, 121
symptoms of, 8
variability in manifestations of, 12
vignettes of, x
Huntington gene, genetic test and, 4
Huntington's chorea, 53–54
Huntington's Disease Society of
    America (HDSA), 249

impulse control, story of Jesse Newsom
    in *Seattle Times,* 211–12
impulsive behavior, 78
insane asylum. *See* asylum(s)
insomnia, 45, 158, 159
interpersonal relationships

family holidays, 177–78
persons with HD, 135
intoxication suspicion
    attorney (HD) with daughter at
        playground, 196–97
    HD confused with, 196, 197–99
    man with HD on Metro bus, 198
    Monica Brewer at jazz club, 198–99
involuntary movements
    Huntington disease, xi, xii, 8
    Tourette syndrome (TS), 17
    see also chorea
IRS (Internal Revenue Service), 157–58
Ith, Ian, 84
It's a Wonderful Life (movie), 191–92

Jamison, Kay Redfield, 18, 155
Jazzercise class, positive attitude, 97
Johnson, David, 4
Jolie, Angelina, 106–7
Jones, E.B. (MD), 196
Jumping Frenchman of Maine, 117
juvenile Huntington disease, 66, 93,
        128–29, 175–76, 256f, 257. *See
        also* children with HD; Princess
        Project

Kennedy, John F., 56
Kesey, Ken, 53, 106–7
King County Jail, 76, 85
King County Superior Court, 75–76, 85
The King's Speech (movie), 188
Koenig, S, 83
Kolata, Gina, 16–17
Kübler-Ross, five stages of grief, 247

lack of awareness, 114–15
LaSpada, A, 251
L-dopa, Parkinson disease, 15–16

legal system, persons with HD, 31–32
life insurance, 26
lobotomy
    frontal, 54–56, 71–72
    transorbital, 54–56
Loman, Linda, 185
long-term care insurance, 26
Lou Gehrig's disease, 16, 47–48, 100
Lowell, Robert, 18, 235–36

mad cow disease, 16–17
magnetic resonance imaging (MRI), 6
    brain, 77, 173–74
    brain of Huntington disease
        patient, 8f
    subdural hematomas, 205–6, 207
malnutrition, 220f
mania, 18, 155, 174
manic, 154–55
manic-depressive illness, 18
marriage
    Beth and Ken (HD), 138
    Carol Carr, husband (HD) and
        family, 139–40
    divorce and HD, 140–41
    Gloria (HD) and Ralph, 137–38
    Kay (HD) and George Wilson,
        143–49, 192
    Margaret, husband (HD) and
        family, 139
    Maria Mendoza decline, 233–34
    Michael (HD) and Marie, 188–92
    persons with HD, 135
    Rachael Morgan (HD) and, 179–80
    Ron Allen (HD) and family, 140–41
Mayo Clinic, 115–16, 222–23
Medicaid, 218
medication, 229, 236, 246. See also
    antidepressants
medium spiny neurons, 7f, 6

melancholia, 53–54
Mendoza, Maria, 233–37
mental disease, 45–46
mental healthcare systems, persons
    with HD, 31–32
mental health professional
    (MHP), 236
mental illness, term, 246
mental institution. See asylum(s)
mental retardation, 3
methadone, 80–81
metro bus diagnosis, 13
mind/body problem, 45–46
mobility, power chair, 147
Moniz, Egas, 54–56
Monroe Prison, George for
    murder, 77, 78
Morgan, Ernest, 214
Morgan, Rachael, 179–82
    common sides of Ben and
        Rachael, 184–85
    marriages of, 179–80
    second son Benjamin, 182–85
morgue, at Western State Hospital,
    59–62
movement disorder, 8
Muncey, Elizabeth, 3
murder, 76, 77, 79–80
Murray, Christopher, 38
muscular dystrophy, 33–34
mutations, 16–17, 125, 257

Nasar, Sylvia, 231
Nash, John, 225–26
National Honor Society, 182, 183
National Institutes of Health (NIH),
    174, 248
National Public Radio, 79–80
Native American reservation
    alcoholism on, 215–16, 217

John and Jerry Greyeagle, 215–18
    tribal mentor on, 216–17, 218
negligence. *See* abuse and neglect
neurogenetics clinic
    clinical team, 33–34
    go-to clinic for HD, 34
Newsom, Jesse, 211–12
Nicholson, Jack, 53, 106–7
Northern State Hospital, 57–58
Northern State Psychiatric Hospital, 37
Nuland, Sherman, 107–8
nursing care, Harold at Willow
    Park, 239–41

obsession, 13, 159, 213–14, 235
obsessive-compulsive behaviors, 213–14
    Parkinson disease, 15–16
    Tourette syndrome (TS), 17
olanzapine, 72
One Flew Over the Cuckoo's Nest
    (film), 106–7
One Flew Over the Cuckoo's Nest
    (Kesey), 53, 106–7
oppositional defiant disorder, 80–81
Oregon State Mental Hospital, 4, 53
O'Sullivan Joseph, 62

parietal lobe, brain pathology in
    AD, 13–14
Paris, Hospital Bicetre, 65–66
Parkinson, James, 15–16
Parkinson disease (PD), x, 6, 77–78,
    213, 248
    neurodegenerative disorder, 15–16
    progression of, 12
    substantia nigra, 7*f*
pathogenic variant, 257
patience, 247
Pelz, Jennifer, 20
penetrance, CAG expansion, 256–57

physical therapy, 246
Pinel, Phillipe, 52, 65–66
pneumonia, 118, 148, 192
police, HD patient taunting, 91
positive approaches
    bowling as outlet for HD, 98
    Carolyn's positive coping skills,
        103–4
    Mary's genetic testing, 95–96
    Mimi's Jazzercise and late onset of
        symptoms, 97
    persons with HD reflecting, 126
    productive older adults with HD,
        121–24, 125
    softball for lawyer Gordon
        Redfield, 98
    Stanley and golden retriever, 99
    teaching for Tim Bennett, 99–101
possession
    battle between good and evil, 227
    Connie and angelic, 228
    Herman Benson and
        diabolical, 227–28
    Jacob and Satan in family, 228–29
    Jason and devil, 227–28
posttraumatic stress disorder
    (PTSD), 123
power chair, mobility of Kay with
    HD, 147
pregnancy, 233–34
    genetic testing during, 168, 169
    termination of, 168, 169
    without genetic testing, 169–70
    preimplantation genetic diagnosis
        (PGD), 169
Princess Project, 129–30
    booklet cover of "Princess in Pink",
        132, 130*f*
    Olympic champion picture by
        Bobbi's classmate, 133*f*

Princess Project (*cont.*)
  pages of "Princess in Pink", 133
  see also children with HD
prion, CJD, 16–17
productive lifestyles, HD in older
    patients, 121–24, 125
proteins, degenerative brain
    diseases, 17
psychosis, 67, 101–2, 107–8, 225–26
psychotherapy, 18, 21, 246
Purple Heart, 121–22
Pussin, Jean-Baptiste, 65–66

Redfield, Gordon, positive attitude
    in HD, 98
Reiswig, Gary, 20, 81
religious life, 43, 44, 227, 228–29
reptilian brain, 75–76
Requiem for a Dream (film), 106–7
research
  brain autopsy for, 60–61, 62
  projects, 248–49
reservation. *See* Native American
    reservation
retirement community, 239–41
Revolutionary Road (film), 106–7
revolving door story, 71
Reynolds, Leonard, 156
Rimer, Sara, 141
Risperdal, 146–47
Robbins, Steven, 165–66
Roberts, Brian, 84, 85, 86
Rossellini, Albert, 38
Rossellini, Victor, 38

Sacks, Oliver, 114–15
St. Elizabeth's Hospital, Washington,
    DC, 54–56
St. John the Evangelist Catholic
    Church, 188

"St. Vitus' dance", 1
Saks, Elyn, 19
  schizophrenia, 6, 45–46, 53–54, 213,
      225–26, 248
  diagnosis of, 79–80
  HD and, 18–19, 231
  patient with HD and, 67
Seattle, Carkeek Park, 83, 84*f*, 86
Seattle Children's Hospital, 128
Seattle Police Department, 83
Seattle Tacoma International
    Airport, 235
Seattle Times (newspaper), 211–12
Seattle VA Medical Center, xi
seizures, 217
senior adults, productive lifestyle and
    HD, 121–24, 125
serotonin, 79–80
shell shock in veterans, 53–54
shelter. *See* homelessness
Simon, Ben, 229–30
Simpson, J, 10
Smith, Frederick, 212
Smith, Sandra, 161–62
social ostracism, 193
Social Security Disability, 104, 117–18,
    164, 184, 217–18
softball, positive attitude in banker
    with, 98
South Dakota Lunatic Asylum, 69–71
speech therapy, 246
stealing, Brian Bachman's arrest for,
    49–50
Steilacoom, Washington, 52–53,
    59–60, 63–64
striatum of basal ganglia, 6, 7*f*
subdural hematoma, 182, 205–6,
    207*f*, 208–9
substantia nigra, Parkinson disease,
    7*f*, 15–16

suicide, 6, 12, 26–27, 101–2,
    212–13
  assisted, 139–40
  end-game strategy, 94
  family members, 139
  by gunshot, 159
  person with HD, 139–40
  thoughts of, 159
Sullivan, Albert
  depression, 105–11
  electroconvulsive therapy (ECT),
    106, 107f, 108, 109–11
  transcranial magnetic stimulation
    (TMS), 109–11
Sumi, Mark, 59–60, 61–62
supportive social network, 93
survivor guilt, 27–28
swallowing, ix
  ALS, 101
  difficulty in, 131, 152–53, 176
  Harold ability in, 241
  therapy, 148, 246
syndrome 5p-, 171

Tabrizi, S, 7
Tacoma General Hospital, 219
TDP-43, FTD and ALS, 17
television, as tranquilizer, 68–69
tertiary syphilis, 53–54
Tet Offensive in Vietnam, 123
Thanksgiving, and social
    interactions, 177
"This American Life" (radio show),
    79–80
Thomas, Bobby, 83
  case in *Seattle Times*
    (newspaper), 84–86
  murdered by roommate,
    84, 85, 86
Thomas, Gordon, 117–19

thousand mile stare, 14, 76
Torrey, E. Fuller, 58
Tourette's syndrome, 17, 117
transcranial magnetic
    stimulation (TMS)
  artist's representation of, 110f
  depression, 109–11
transorbital leucotomy, 54–56
transport, ceiling railway system,
    148–49
Tuke, William, 52

UCLA, 19
University Hospital genetics lab, 90
University Medical Center
    (Seattle), 201–2
University of Iowa, 179–80
University of Washington, 33–34, 35,
    143–44, 182
Urbach-Wiethe, 66–67

VanDuser, William and Evelyn, 171–76
  adopting Vicki (HD), 171–73
  discovering Vicki's HD in
    family, 173–74
  raising Vicki's son Phillip, 174,
    175–76
variants, 257
Veterans Affairs (VA) Hospital, 121–22,
    187–88
Veterans Affairs (VA) Medical
    Centers, 123
Veterans Affairs (VA) veteran, 151–52
violence, 101–2
  George murdering roommate, 76
  Phineas Gage, 78–79

Washington (state)
  "Death with Dignity" law, 47–48
  Fort Steilacoom, 52–53, 59–60

Washington State Hospital, HD
    patients, 57–58, 64–69
Washington State Penitentiary, Walla
    Walla, WA, 34, 35–36, 78, 245
Western State Hospital (WSH), 62, 91,
    106–7, 212–13, 225–26
    asylum museum and cemetery, 71–72
    deinstitutionalization and, 57–58
    history of, 52–53
    interactions with staff at, 63–64
    meeting HD patients at, 64–71
    morgue at, 59–62
West Riding Pauper Lunatic
    Asylum, 52
Wexler, Alice, 10
Wexler, Nancy, 4
Williams, Tennessee, 54–56
Williams, William Carlos, xii, xii
Willow Park retirement
    community, 239–41

Wilson, George, 141
    aiding food swallowing for Kay, 148
    attending church, 147
    Kay's father with HD in Arizona
        prison, 144
    Kay's speech with HD, 147
    marriage to Kay (with HD),
        143–49
    medication for Kay, 146–47
    mobility for Kay, 147
    therapy for Kay's behavior, 145–46
    transport apparatus for Kay, 148–49
Wilson, George and Kay, 143–49
Wilson, Ward, 154–55, 156–57, 213
World War I, 55
World War II, 123, 188

X-rays, 201–2, 203, 206

Zen, 202–3